ASPIRIN THERAPY

ASPIRIN THERAPY

Paul E. Schindler, Jr.

Foreword by William S. Fields, M.D.

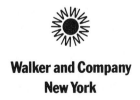

Walker and Company
New York

To Carol Ann Franz and Paul and Mari Schindler, my parents

First published in the United States of America
in 1978 by the Walker Publishing Company, Inc.
Published simultaneously in Canada by Beaverbooks,
Limited, Pickering, Ontario
ISBN: 0-8027-0565-0
Library of Congress Catalog Card Number: 76-56688
Printed in the United States of America
10 9 8 7 6 5 4 3 2 1

Contents

Acknowledgments

No book results from the efforts of a single person, despite the fact that the author's work is often considered solitary. First, my thanks to Carol Ann Franz, whose emotional and financial support made easier the difficult task of writing this book. Secondly, my thanks to Edwin Diamond of MIT, my journalism professor and good friend, who recommended me for the job of writing this book and who gave much sound advice. Finally, my thanks go to my parents who raised me to believe I could do anything I wanted to do.

Also instrumental in the completion of this volume were: Richard K. Winslow, of Walker and Company, who shepherded the manuscript through its drafts; Hershel Jick, M.D., who provided advice and assistance; William Brooks of Sterling Drug and Terry Kelley of Upjohn who arranged interviews; Barb Moore, John Hanzel and Norman Sandler, who told me I could do it; Elizabeth Wild for translation; my employers, UPI and Bank of America, for their understanding, particularly the bank's public information manager Raymond V. Toman; and all those I interviewed and all the medical researchers whose papers I have read, without whose work mine would not exist.

Special thanks to Dr. William S. Fields for writing the foreword. Where I am correct, I stand on the shoulders of giants; where I have erred, the responsibility is mine alone.

Foreword

This volume is dedicated to focusing public attention on a truly remarkable pharmaceutical agent which has been around for eighty years. This drug has been so widely used and its easy availability taken so much for granted that its mode of action has been largely overlooked. In the United States, at least, the old adage "Go home, take two aspirin, go to bed, and call me in the morning" has become so embedded in public consciousness that it has become difficult for a physician to convince his patients that the recently discovered virtues of such a commonplace medication may have a profound impact on the treatment of serious national health problems.

There is little doubt that the information contained herein will contribute immeasurably to the general awareness of significant properties which always have been present inside the "little white tablet" and even now are not completely understood. The book presents a carefully considered and accurate reflection of the current state of our knowledge about aspirin and the research into its pharmacologic mechanisms and clinical applications.

One cannot consider the bright new prospects for this old "friend" without contemplating the difficulties which would have undoubtedly been encountered had it arrived on the scene in the

United States in 1977 instead of 1897. In a recently completed large, multicentered clinical trial, it was found necessary to file an IND (Investigational New Drug) application with the Food and Drug Administration to acquire a number for aspirin before starting, even though this trial was federally sponsored. This regulation arises from the clear statement in public law requiring that any pharmaceutical agent approved for use in one medical context must be considered investigational and nonapproved when prescribed in another. Although consumer protection is a very important element in the introduction of new drugs, it seems over-zealous on the part of the bureaucracy to extend this prerequisite to the study of a drug for which the over-the-counter approved daily dose is 12 five-grain tablets (3.9 grams) and that suggested for the controlled trial only four tablets (1.3 grams). Furthermore, if one considers that many new drugs are available to physicians and their patients in Canada, Mexico and western Europe months or even years before they are approved, much less marketed, in the United States, it is certainly conceivable that aspirin as a new drug might be among them.

Not only is aspirin a remarkably effective drug, but it is surprisingly free of toxic side effects when taken in an approved dosage. However, as with all substances that may be taken by mouth, rare individuals will be encountered who have an intolerance for the drug and taking even one tablet may be hazardous. In addition, there are those who have medical conditions such as bleeding disorders for whom aspirin use would be ill-advised. The book's author has carefully weighed the "risk-benefit ratio" and concluded that when one considers the importance of potential new benefits, particularly those related to cardiovascular disease, the evidence is heavily in favor of efficacy as well as safety. He would, however, be the first to emphasize that aspirin used on a regular and continuing basis be taken only on the advice of one's physician.

Mr. Schindler is to be congratulated for taking an everyday event and creating from it an exciting story.

—WILLIAM S. FIELDS, M.D.

1
Aspirin in Perspective

Aspirin is better than you think. It deserves the designation "marvel."

The world's best-selling medical substance, aspirin, was first sold in 1899. Yet its method of operation was unknown until recently, and it will be several more years before its potentially most significant effect will be proven or disproven. If aspirin is not a marvel—a substance of wonder whose story has been long in unfolding—it is the closest thing yet discovered.

Can aspirin reduce the incidence of heart attack and stroke, the most common disease causes of death in the industrialized world? Studies now underway attempt to answer the question, but researchers already know regular aspirin users appear to have fewer heart attacks than persons who seldom take aspirin. In the search for a definitive answer results are not expected until 1980.

In the meantime, most impressions of aspirin are being formed by oft-distorted, competitive pain-relief-product advertising, much of which stresses infrequent, insignificant side effects. Presently, aspirin is effective, inexpensive, and safe for treatment of pain, fever, and inflammation. Someday, aspirin could be proven effective, safe, and inexpensive for heart-attack prevention.

A running debate on aspirin's effectiveness in reducing heart-attack risk has been carried on in medical journals for twenty-one years, ever since California physician Dr. Lawrence L. Craven reported fewer heart attacks among his patients who took aspirin. The results of three recent studies, indicating reduced heart-attack risk among aspirin-takers, encouraged the federal government to launch a $17 million program to test aspirin's ability to prevent a subsequent heart attack in those who have already survived an initial attack.

The federal study was also encouraged by recent breakthroughs in the effort to understand how aspirin works in the human body. Until the last few years, aspirin's mode of action was only dimly understood. This understanding has increased greatly, thanks to increased research into hormonelike substances called prostaglandins. Aspirin appears to achieve its reduction of pain, fever, and inflammation mostly by suppression of the body's natural manufacture of prostaglandins (PGs). Since PGs aid in clot formation, and clots play a role in heart attacks and strokes, reduction of the PG level in the body may decrease clot formation and thus reduce the incidence of these two diseases.

As a rule, however, the story of how aspirin works, or the possibility it may reduce heart-attack risk, are reported less often than its rare side effects, which are routinely touted in the multi-million-dollar advertising campaigns of pain-relief products that purport to be an improvement over aspirin. Yet the risks of taking aspirin are likely to be slim indeed compared with its proven benefits. At normal dose levels, aspirin is exceedingly useful and remarkably safe.

Aspirin's utility may be indicated by its ubiquity. In the United States alone, aspirin is consumed at a rate of 100 tablets per citizen per year; enough aspirin to create a stack bigger than New York City's World Trade Center. Sales of aspirin-based products in the United States during 1975 amounted to $700 million. Yet the cost to the consumer of one tablet of straight aspirin—with all its diversity of uses—was little more than a cent.

Aspirin-taking is widespread. About 15 percent of the population—33 million Americans—take aspirin once a week or more. Of that group, 40 percent take aspirin four times a week or more. Aspirin daily doses may vary from one 80-milligram tablet for a child to twenty 325-milligram tablets for an adult suffering from arthritis.

Heart-Attack Prevention

Why did it take seventy-eight years for researchers to notice a relationship between the most popular medicine and the most common cause of death? Naturally, the great complexity of factors that contribute to heart-attack risk obscure the role of any one drug. Besides, it *has* been decades since a few doctors noticed that regular aspirin-taking seemed to reduce heart-attack risk. But scientific efforts to prove the relationship are only a few years old and remain several years from completion. Additionally, it was not until the 1970s that understanding of aspirin's mode of action was sufficient to provide an acceptable explanation of such risk reduction.

During the last five years, research into the causes of heart attacks and strokes, and into aspirin's operation, has yielded surprising results. The two diseases may result from a particular malfunction of the blood-clotting system, which aspirin is especially suited to prevent. The public has been informed of the progress in discovering the causes of heart attacks; but aspirin's protective capability has remained largely unexplained because, until recently, it was unknown.

The first physician to publish his finding of an aspirin–heart-attack relationship was the late Dr. Lawrence L. Craven of Glendale, California. After some chance observations in the late 1940s, he became convinced by 1950 that regular aspirin-takers had fewer heart attacks. In 1956, he reported on a ten-year study of 8,000 aspirin-taking men. None had suffered a heart attack or stroke, Craven said. Medical scientists discounted Craven's study because of the informal manner in which it was conducted. Nevertheless, it remained a provocative report that partially inspired later and more rigorous investigations.

Since then, however, at least three major studies of the frequency of heart attacks and one study of strokes among persons regularly taking aspirin have yielded encouraging results: the risk of either disease appeared to be less for aspirin-takers than for non-aspirin-takers.

One 1976 U.S. study of 179 stroke victims showed a 30 percent drop in second strokes among aspirin-takers in various geographic areas. A 1974 study of 18,000 patients in Boston-area hospitals showed heart-attack victims were at least twice as likely to be infrequent aspirin-takers as persons with similar characteristics who had not had a heart attack. In a 1974 British study, the death rate among 566 aspirin-takers with one heart attack was less than that among 560 persons not taking aspirin regularly. A 1975 study of 1,529 Americans showed a 30 percent reduction in the death rate after one heart attack among those who took aspirin.

These results have been called "tantalizing," "provocative," and "promising" by medical researchers. The studies have not yet been called "conclusive," but some were too short or involved too few people to insure results caused by aspirin-taking, rather than chance. One study was "retrospective," asking heart-attack victims about prior drug use. "Prospective" studies, those that follow a patient's drug use prior to an attack, are generally considered more meaningful.

In order to obtain conclusive evidence of a relationship between aspirin and heart-attack risk, researchers must conduct prospective studies under strict control, using modern methods, involving large numbers of people for long periods of time. Such studies are expensive.

Already underway is one such nationwide study, comparing the effect of daily aspirin doses with treatment by an inert sugar pill. The National Heart, Lung and Blood Institute (NHLBI), a federal agency, is conducting the three-year, 4,500-participant study among persons who have had one heart attack. The numbers of patients and length of examination needed to obtain statistically reliable results are reduced by limiting the study to previous victims, who are five times as likely as the general population to die or have an attack during a given period of time. (See Chapter 7.)

4

The $17 million Aspirin Myocardial Infarction Study (*myocardial infarction* is the medical term for heart attack) compares the effect of three aspirin tablets a day with that of three identical-looking sugar pills. The AMIS results, expected in 1980, could be "really profound," according to the federal official who supervises the project, Dr. William Friedewald, medical officer of the NHLBI Clinical Trials Branch.

Indeed, if aspirin, a safe, inexpensive drug, is also proven effective for reducing the risk of heart attack and stroke, this could spark a revolution in medical care. Millions of persons, especially those whose lifestyle and family history mark them as prime heart-attack candidates, may be able to cut their chances of premature death from these two diseases with regular aspirin doses.

Aspirin Therapy?

Even before the recent studies, Dr. Lee Wood, now a blood specialist in California, proposed aspirin therapy to reduce heart-attack risk. In 1972, he wrote the eminent British medical journal *Lancet*, suggesting that one aspirin tablet per day be prescribed for men over twenty and women over forty to reduce their risk of heart attack.

Wood claims the proposed regimen has small risks and enormous potential benefits. But his recommendation was adopted by only a few physicians, who generally believe all drug-taking involves risk, which must be balanced by substantial, proven benefits. As a whole, the medical profession awaits clearer proof of the benefits of aspirin with respect to heart attacks and strokes before recommending it as Dr. Wood does.

The operating head of the Aspirin Myocardial Infarction Study is Dr. James Schoenberger of St. Luke's Hospital in Chicago. He heads the AMIS steering committee, guiding its analysis of the relationship between aspirin and heart-attack risk. Schoenberger emphatically opposes general aspirin-taking to reduce heart-attack risk before his and other studies are completed. "It would be a disaster if the public began to take aspirin willy-nilly, day in and day out, before we know all the benefits and risks," he said.

Both Wood and Schoenberger have a point. They both believe that taking aspirin to reduce the risk of heart attack is a matter of balancing risks and benefits. Wood believes there is already enough evidence of a low-risk level to make uncertain benefits seem promising. Schoenberger does not believe present, haphazard aspirin-taking patterns predict the effects of regular, long-term low doses. The evidence favors Wood. Aspirin's risks are known, and low. The benefits, perhaps high, are still being uncovered.

Aspirin's Operation

Prostaglandins (PGs), powerful regulators of body chemistry, are among the most widely investigated medical substances of the 1970's—and are the source of aspirin's major effects. Aspirin apparently works by supressing natural production of PGs, a relationship which remained undiscovered until laboratory techniques and equipment became sufficently refined to detect it, an event of the 1970's.

Aspirin's power and wide-ranging effects result from the strength and effect of PGs, the most powerful known chemical the body produces; significant effects can be caused by less than one-ten-billionth of an ounce. PGs perform a control function in reproduction and disease-fighting systems; they may encourage spontaneous miscarriages or cancer's symptoms. Aspirin effectively controls PGs, so it may in turn control PG-triggered conditions. As PG research expands to a number of bodily systems, aspirin's role is also expected to expand.

Acetylsalicylic acid, ASA, aspirin or $C_9H_8O_4$ (nine carbon atoms, eight hydrogen atoms and four oxygen atoms), in doses as small as a single tablet, can prevent PG synthesis throughout the body. Although some cells recover in minutes, platelets (a type of blood cell) can never again make PGs after exposure to aspirin; these cells are replaced in an average of five days.

Clotting and "hardening of the arteries," or atherosclerosis, both involve PG release by platelets and both contribute to heart attacks and strokes. Thus, theoretically, aspirin's prevention of PG release by platelets could reduce the incidence of the diseases.

The PG role in pain, fever, and inflammation is no longer theoretical, according to Britain's Dr. John R. Vane, one of the discoverers of the PG-aspirin link. All three symptoms are reduced, either in the presence of aspirin or the absence of PGs, he says, leaving only "a few pockets of resistance" to the theory that PG-suppression explains aspirin's effects.

The conditions for which aspirin is suggested or avoided may change as more physicians accept this explanation of its operation. Conditions caused by excess PGs, whether or not they involve overt pain, fever, and inflammation, will be treated with aspirin. Conditions prolonged by a lack of PGs will have to be treated with some other drug. In short, physicians will more precisely predict which illnesses will respond to aspirin treatment.

Wide Use

Shortly after it was introduced, aspirin became the world's most widely used medicine, because it quickly proved to be relatively safe, effective for a wide range of symptoms and inexpensive.

Aspirin's safety is indicated by the low number of poisoning cases it is involved in, despite its availability and wide use. If aspirin were not relatively safe at normal doses, epidemics of aspirin poisoning would be reported daily. There are no such epidemics, so there must be widespread tolerance for the drug—when taken as directed by the label or a doctor.

Aspirin is relatively inexpensive, both compared with other pain relievers and to drugs in general. A single two-tablet dose of aspirin costs no more than two cents; a day's maximum dosage costs less than a quarter. Other pain relievers are often twice and even ten times as expensive as aspirin; other drugs cost hundreds of times as much.

Since other pain relievers and other drugs have been developed in an effort to supplant aspirin, it has not held its reputation because of a lack of competition. Although not all drugs are intended for the same purposes as aspirin, the extent of drug research is shown by the existence of 1,000 drugs now in common usage. There are 40 new drugs developed each year; roughly a similar number fall into disuse and become obsolete annually. Some 90 percent of the drugs available today were unknown in 1950; half had not been developed by 1960. Aspirin is one of a handful of drugs that has been in constant, high-volume use for more than fifty years.

Most of aspirin's effects are palliative, or symptom-relieving, rather than cause-relieving. One exception—and it is a major exception—is arthritis, in which inflammation is both a symptom and a cause. Another possible exception may be heart attacks and strokes.

Aspirin's major palliative effects have been proven beyond reasonable doubt during seventy-eight years of usage. There is no better drug for mild cases of pain, fever, and inflammation.

Both the Food and Drug Administration and the American Medical Association have recognized aspirin's utility for treatment of these symptoms. The FDA's advisory panel on non-prescription pain relievers and fever reducers found aspirin to be one of only six substances available without prescription that are safe and effective for pain and fever. *Drug Evaluations,* an AMA guide, suggests aspirin for headache, fever and bone and muscle pain. The AMA also recommends doctors try aspirin first when treating inflammation caused by most forms of arthritis, and that they use other, more expensive drugs only when aspirin fails.

Aspirin can even relieve the pain of childbirth, a use to which it and its chemical cousins have been put since the time of Hippocrates, several hundred years B.C.

What It Is

Substances derived from plants have been used to relieve pain for thousands of years; today's aspirin is derived from petroleum or coal tar. Aspirin manufacturing starts with the production of salicylic acid (SA) from a light petroleum fraction. The SA undergoes a process known as acetylation (described in Chapter 2) and becomes acetylsalicylic acid, or aspirin.

Salicin, a close but weak relative of ASA, was the first form of aspirin, extracted from the bark and leaves of the willow tree and swallowed as a general pain killer. It was not until the early 1800s that European scientists discovered salicin was most concentrated in the "spirea" family of plants.

The spireas include Queen of the Prarie (Queen of the Meadow in Europe), Bridal Wreath, Meadowsweet, and Hardhack —all thin, woody shrubs of the rose family. In addition to being members of the spirea family, the "queens" are also classified as perennial herbs. Pure salicin was first extracted in quantity from members of this plant family. Other shrubs, grasses, and trees contain small amounts of salicin, while trace amounts of it are found in oranges, apples, and grapes.

Aspirin Products

The United States is one of the few countries in the world in which the word "aspirin" refers to all forms of ASA, no matter who manufactured it. In seventy other countries, including Germany, Austria, Denmark, Belgium, Brazil, and Chile, the word "aspirin" is a trademark, is spelled with a capital A and can be used only by Bayer AG of Leverkusen, West Germany, the original manufacturer. In the United States, the name Bayer belongs to Sterling Drug Inc., which lost a court suit to defend the aspirin trademark. Sterling holds both the Bayer name and the "Aspirin" trademark in Canada.

Thus, in the United States, all acetylsalicylic acid is called "aspirin." But "aspirin" is often avoided in product names, relegating the word to ingredient-list fine-print. Thus, although Anacin and Bufferin consist primarily of aspirin, many people are unaware of their contents, despite the label. This is not surprising; the New

York Pharmacology Society found 85 percent of those surveyed either did not read or did not understand the labels of over-the-counter drugs they used.

The common names for plain aspirin include acetylsalicylic acid, ASA, and ASA, U.S.P. (for United States Pharmacopeia). The initials USP indicate the aspirin claims to meet minimum product standards of the pharmaceutical industry. Another set of initials, APC, causes some confusion. APC, manufactured by several firms, is often mistaken for plain aspirin. It is actually a combination product, containing aspirin, phenacetin, and caffeine.

Plain aspirin brands, which had a retail value of $144 million in 1975, include best-sellers Bayer and St. Joseph's.

Combination products, with a sales volume of $437 million, were led by Anacin, Bufferin, and Excedrin. These products consist mostly of aspirin.

Most aspirin substitutes, on which the public spent $73 million in 1975, were based on the chemical acetaminophen. The most popular brand is Tylenol; other brand names include Datril, Liquiprin, and Tempra.

When combined with the $93.9 million spent on arthritis medicines, most of which are aspirin or aspirin-based, the total U.S. expenditure for pain relievers in 1975 amounted to more than $700 million. About 90 percent of the total was spent for aspirin products!

How Much? Who Takes It?

All the spirea plants in the United States would come nowhere near meeting the demand for aspirin in this country every year. If placed in a single stack, the annual supply of aspirin tablets would reach the moon. There are 14 million doctors' recommendations for aspirin each year, according to Sterling Drug, makers of Bayer. All told, U.S. consumption amounts to more than 25 million tons of aspirin, sold under thousands of brand names.

Although mountains of aspirin are consumed by those with fevers and headaches, half of the 22 billion aspirin tablets taken annually are taken by arthritics, primarily the elderly.

Risks

Aspirin is widely misunderstood, in part because of advertising pitches that have left many people with the impression it is a drug to be avoided. On balanced consideration, this is incorrect.

At normal doses, nearly every widely used medical substance causes more side effects, more often, than aspirin. A conservative estimate of side effects is that 5 percent of the public has any noticeable reaction to aspirin. Put another way, 95 out of 100 persons who take aspirin do not even suffer so minor a side effect as heartburn after taking the drug.

There are a very few people who should avoid aspirin: a few thousand in the United States take drugs that would interact adversely; perhaps one person in 25,000 is allergic to aspirin. Drug interaction and allergy are not considerations for most people. Additionally, in line with the general advice against drug use during pregnancy, an FDA advisory panel has suggested women avoid aspirin during the last three months of pregnancy unless it is taken under a doctor's supervision.

Drug interaction and allergy are no more difficult to determine than pregnancy, so knowing when to avoid aspirin is easy. If a person is allergic, one tablet usually indiciates the problem, by causing swollen lips and eyelids. If other drugs pose the threat of interaction, the prescribing physician will know.

Because aspirin is generally palliative, not curative, its long-term use without the supervision of a physician is undesirable. Continuing pain, fever, or inflammation may indicate a serious disease; needed medical attention may be delayed if the symptoms are masked by aspirin. Any pain, however minor, which continues for weeks may be serious and should not be self-treated.

Some other risks commonly associated with aspirin are less serious than generally believed. Some are outright nonexistent. Dan-

11

gerous stomach bleeding is *not* the result of every dose of aspirin. Tolerance is *not* developed after repeated doses. Although some non-aspirin pain relievers advertise that "millions" should not take aspirin, there is *no* firm evidence to support this claim.

Stomach bleeding from aspirin is less serious than most persons realize. Most people bleed an unnoticed and medically insignificant half-teaspoon of blood from the stomach every day. Tests show a daily dose of twelve tablets increases the total to one and a half teaspoons, an amount that can only be detected with laboratory tests and is still medically insignificant.

Advertising may be the source of some public misunderstanding. Pain-reliever advertising has focused for years on the hazards of aspirin without additives; more recently, non-aspirin products have stressed the "risks" of aspirin products in general.

Both of these points are wildly exaggerated. Additives now available make no detectable difference for the vast majority of persons who take aspirin. Yet advertising creates the illusion of greatly increased incidence of side effects with plain aspirin.

For an even larger majority, non-aspirin pain relievers like Tylenol and Datril (both based on acetaminophen) are unnecessary. They are probably as effective as aspirin for pain, but acetaminophen products are ineffective for inflammation and may be more hazardous. Despite advertising to the contrary, they are certainly *not* safer than aspirin.

Although physicians prefer plain aspirin to reduce pain, fever, and inflammation, multi-ingredient products and aspirin substitutes outsell any aspirin brand; Tylenol (substitute) is the best seller, followed by Anacin (multi-ingredient). Medical evidence does not support such a sales advantage; neither does balancing risks and benefits. Anacin and Tylenol must be presumed to have attained their position via advertising.

On Balance

Whenever medical authorities have balanced the risks and benefits of aspirin, benefits have predominated, from its 1899 discovery in

Germany to its recent review by the FDA. Bayer AG found it safe in the first place; the FDA advisory panel on pain relievers balanced seventy-eight years of reports to favor aspirin's continued use.

The highly regarded *New England Journal of Medicine* expressed similar sentiments in a recent editorial, which said, "Seen from a broad perspective, aspirin is probably the world's most useful analgesic [pain reliever]." When minor pain is the symptom, aspirin is the first drug to try, according to the AMA's desktop drug reference, *Drug Evaluations*.

Aspirin benefits clearly outweigh risks for short-term low-dosage treatment of non-recurring pain, fever, and inflammation. The risk-benefit ratio improves further if persons who should not take aspirin (those allergic to it, or taking drugs that interact, among others) are excluded.

The risk-benefit ratio is not yet so clearly defined for aspirin-taking to reduce heart-attack risk, but appears promising. And, as science comes to better understand prostaglandins, aspirin—which controls PGs—will no doubt be taken even more widely than is now the case.

If any drug in the modern medicine chest is a marvel, it is aspirin.

2

Buying Aspirin and Taking It

Pain, fever, and inflammation are the symptoms that aspirin relieves best. Most people take aspirin because it is inexpensive, safe, and effective for these common complaints.

Most mild pain occurs during everyday headaches, for which aspirin is the best treatment. Severe headaches are another matter —they may indicate a serious disorder.

Fever, from the flu or the common cold, is a minor aid to the body as it fights infection, but a major source of discomfort to the victim. Physicians use aspirin to relieve the discomfort, since it is the best non-prescription fever reducer.

Inflammation is the most debilitating symptom of arthritis; but its characteristic symptoms of red, swollen, and partially immobile joints are relieved by aspirin, which restores mobility and reduces pain, providing arthritics a temporary respite from their discomfort.

While aspirin is most commonly taken for the symptoms of headache, flu, colds, and arthritis, it will also relieve the same unpleasant symptoms when they occur during countless other diseases and ailments.

15

How to Take Aspirin

Most people think aspirin-taking is uncomplicated, and they are usually right. But hints on how to take it can provide faster and longer-lasting relief, at somewhat lower cost and with less chance of side effects.

There are several techniques of aspirin-taking that minimize the chances of stomach upset. Aspirin should always be taken with a liquid. If it is taken "dry," the tablets disintegrate more slowly in the stomach. This delays their effectiveness and increases the chances of an undissolved particle irritating the stomach lining.

The same goal—to decrease irritation by decreasing dissolving time—leads some physicians to recommend chewing aspirin tablets, then drinking a glass of water. For those who cannot stand the taste of aspirin, the alternative is to push the tablets into a milk-filled mouth, then chew and swallow.

If speedy effectiveness is desired, the least expensive way to achieve it with regular aspirin tablets is to chew them, then drink a glass of lukewarm water. The water may be flavored with honey or sugar to make the taste less unpleasant.

When slow effectiveness over a period of time is desired, the American Medical Association publication *Drug Evaluations* recommends eating or drinking prior to taking aspirin, since the dissolved drug leaves a full intestinal tract more slowly than an empty one.

Those who must take aspirin for long periods of time should be wary of even the slight increased stomach bleeding aspirin sometimes causes. The American Pharmaceutical Association's *Handbook of Non-Prescription Drugs* suggests use of an antacid, or acid-neutralizing, drug along with aspirin. Products that combine antacids with aspirin do not contain enough antacid to neutralize fully the acid in their aspirin, the APHA found. But separate pill or liquid antacids can reduce stomach bleeding to near zero.

An antacid that will be used frequently should be "non-absorbable," such as Di-Gel, Maalox, or Mylanta, rather than absorbable, such as Rolaids, Tums or Alka-Seltzer. Pharmacists can advise which antacids are non-absorbable. About one tablespoon of the liquid form of the three non-absorbable antacids mentioned neutralizes the acid in two aspirin tablets.

How Often, How Much

Unless otherwise directed by a physician, an adult should take no more than two 325 milligram (5 grain) aspirin tablets every four hours. Daily intake should be limited to ten tablets. For headache pain, aspirin reaches its peak efficiency in about two hours, then decreases slowly. For fever relief, aspirin's effect peaks after three hours, then decreases.

The two tablets/four hours dosage schedule maximizes benefits while minimizing risks. Larger quantities improve relief slightly but may greatly increase side effects. More frequent doses could increase aspirin in the blood to dangerous levels; it takes an average of four hours for most aspirin and aspirin by-products to leave the blood (and forty-eight hours to leave the body, through the kidneys by urination).

When Not to Take Aspirin

There are five factors that might lead to a decision to avoid taking aspirin:

1. No need. Aspirin is not usually needed for mild pain, which will stop by itself without any treatment.
2. Recurring symptoms. If pain, fever, and inflammation persist, taking aspirin will only "mask" these symptoms, which can indicate a serious underlying problem.
3. Permanent conditions. Persons with ulcers and hemophilia, as well as the very few persons who are allergic to aspirin, should not take it.
4. Temporary conditions. Women in the last three

17

months of pregnancy and persons planning to undergo major surgery should avoid aspirin (unless a physician recommends otherwise).

5. Drug interactions. There are certain drugs that do not work properly, or cause side effects, when taken with aspirin.

Aspirin can mask the severity of an illness and delay adequate medical care, leaving an aspirin-taker to suddenly discover a major medical problem developed while early warning symptoms were covered up by the drug. The necessary precaution is straightforward: any symptom that recurs for weeks should be brought to a doctor's attention.

This masking and delayed-care syndrome can be especially dangerous in undiagnosed cases of arthritis, whose symptoms are very effectively controlled by aspirin. This danger led a prestigious advisory panel of the Food and Drug Administration to warn against aspirin self-treatment if arthritis is suspected. The panel points out there is a risk of irreversible damage to joints and tissue if aspirin is used without medical supervision.

To reduce self-treatment, the FDA panel has proposed a ban on the use of the word "arthritis" in the names of some pain relievers. These products generally contain larger than normal amounts of aspirin. Tablets that contain twice as much aspirin each cut in half the number of separate tablets arthritics must take to ingest the same weight of aspirin. Although such products may ease the treatment of arthritis, the FDA panel believes they encourage aspirin-taking without a physician's advice.

Permanent Conditions

Ulcers, hemophilia, and aspirin intolerance are permanent physical conditions that preclude aspirin taking. All are relatively rare, and once they have been diagnosed, the patient must avoid aspirin in all forms.

Persons with serious stomach problems, especially ulcers, should avoid taking aspirin. Ulcers are breaks in the stomach or intestine lining that expose the delicate tissue underneath. Bits of aspirin that have not fully dissolved can enlarge such breaks, or encourage the lining to flake off entirely.

If ulcers are already present, they may bleed more after aspirin ingestion, because aspirin slightly increases a person's bleeding time.

Those who cannot tolerate aspirin are commonly said to suffer from "aspirin allergy" or "aspirin asthma." Once this intolerance is diagnosed, usually after a sudden attack of wheezing following aspirin ingestion, the drug is avoided. Physicians can now perform tests to discover if a person is aspirin intolerant. In most instances, such persons have a history of asthma.

On rare occasions, a person who has never had asthma or adverse reactions to aspirin may suddenly become intolerant late in life. Again, once this rare syndrome has manifested itself, control is simply a matter of avoiding aspirin and aspirin-containing products.

Hemophiliacs, and others with blood-clotting disorders, should not take aspirin. It can worsen their condition. Hemophiliacs have a clotting system that is one-third inoperative—they still have some protection against bleeding. Aspirin further weakens the remaining two-thirds of the hemophiliac's clotting mechanism. As a result, hemophiliacs can suffer severe internal bleeding if they receive even a minor blow or injury after taking aspirin.

Temporary Physical Conditions

Pregnancy and upcoming surgery are two temporary situations in which aspirin-taking without a physician's advice is not a good idea. Aspirin may still be taken; in some cases it may be prescribed. But during these conditions, caution is wise.

Labor time and delivery difficulties may be increased in women who take aspirin prior to giving birth. In addition, if they have aspirin in their bodies, both mother and child will experience slightly greater bleeding time, which can add to the hazards of a complicated delivery. Presently, the FDA is considering a label warning for aspirin products, advising against aspirin-taking during the last three months of pregnancy, without a doctor's advice.

Aspirin is sometimes prescribed prior to surgery to reduce the incidence of clots (see Chapter 7) before operations on older persons, or preceeding lower limb operations, when clots are a common side effect.

Typically, doctors advise against aspirin before most surgery. Aspirin's reduction of blood clotting, the very process that holds such promise in heart-attack reduction, can spell trouble in complicated operations. Surgery puts a great load on the clotting mechanism that, obviously, should be in top condition prior to a major operation. If impaired clotting is feared, the doctor will usually suggest aspirin avoidance for two weeks before surgery (the time it takes the clotting effect to wear off).

Drug Interactions

In general, a drug is any chemical agent that affects living matter. In particular, the U.S. Food and Drug Administration defines a drug as a substance introduced into the body to diagnose, treat, or prevent illness.

Under the first definition, alcohol and nicotine are the world's most widely used drugs. Under the second definition, aspirin is the most widely used drug. To maintain the distinction, aspirin is referred to here as the most widely used medical substance.

If two drugs, taken simultaneously or sequentially, interfere with each others' operation, they are said to interact. Aspirin interacts with many drugs, both prescription and non-prescription (also known as over-the-counter or OTC).

Alcohol is one "drug" with which aspirin reacts adversely. Consumption of alcohol makes the stomach sensitive to irritation for as long as twelve hours. Aspirin taken during this period is more likely to cause stomach bleeding or upset. Thus, taking aspirin for hangovers is a dubious proposition.

Another dubious proposition is attempted reduction of cold symptoms with simultaneous use of aspirin and large doses of vitamin C—500 milligrams per hour in some cases. Vitamin C is not usually categorized as a drug, but in such doses its effects can be as powerful as some drugs. When taken in large doses, vitamin C interacts with aspirin. Under normal conditions, both vitamin C and aspirin are eliminated from the bloodstream at a steady pace. When both drugs are present, the elimination of vitamin C takes place more quickly, that of aspirin more slowly. As a result, the vitamin C is less effective, while the aspirin may build up to near-toxic levels, since it is not half-eliminated when the next dose is taken, four hours later, as is normally the case.

A common drug interaction involves taking unprescribed aspirin while being treated with an anti-arthritic drug. Doctors sometimes prescribe aspirin and other anti-arthritic drugs together. Under this regimen, the dose of each drug can be lowered in order to reduce the side effects of both. Persons taking anti-arthritic drugs should not take additional aspirin without first consulting their physician.

Some widely used anti-arthritic drugs are Azolid, Butazolidin, Indocin, Sterazolidin, Tandearil, and many drugs containing cortisone or cortisone derivatives.

A much less common interaction occurs when aspirin is taken during treatment with anti-clotting medicine, usually administered after a first heart-attack. Such drugs as Athrombin-K, Coumadin, Panwarfin, Dicumarol and Sintrom, among others, popularly known as "blood-thinners," reduce the blood's ability to clot. So does aspirin. Simultaneous use can lead to severe internal and external bleeding.

Drugs used to lower the body's uric acid level, usually to control gout, interact with aspirin. In small doses, aspirin increases uric acid levels, while in large doses it reduces them and causes side effects. Although once used as a gout treatment, aspirin has been replaced by more effective drugs, such as Anturane and Benemid, which should not be taken simultaneously with aspirin.

21

Avoiding Aspirin

Avoiding aspirin can be a difficult task: it is everywhere, from the Apollo spacecraft medicine kit to the family medicine chest. The Food and Drug Administration says aspirin and aspirin-based products are sold under 50,000 trade names, some of which do not clearly indicate that aspirin is an ingredient.

Aspirin is so common many people do not think of it as a drug. General practitioners find they get quite different answers to the question, "taking any medicines" and "taking any aspirin?"

One case history involved a Houston woman who took twenty-five aspirin tablets a day during her pregnancy. "If I'd known aspirin was a drug, I wouldn't have taken it," she said. Hers is an extreme case.

But aspirin-taking is also ignored in less extreme cases. The Red Cross surveyed randomly selected blood donors across the United States, asking if they had taken aspirin in the last week. Thirty percent said they had; yet blood tests on the others revealed that another 11 percent of them had chemical traces indicating aspirin ingestion within the week.

Such unadmitted aspirin-taking may not be solely the result of poor memory, since aspirin is sold under so many names. But whether the label says "ASA" or "cold medicine," if it contains aspirin, it has the same effect on the body.

Reading the label clears up most content questions, but even general scientific knowledge is no guarantee of label understanding.

One prominent electrical engineer tells of suffering from hives during colds for years. He did not attribute them to aspirin until his hives broke out during a bout with several headaches. "It must have been the aspirin, so I switched to Bufferin," he said. The change of name cleared up the hives, perhaps by power of suggestion, but not through chemical effect. Bufferin is a trade name for aspirin, with some antacid added.

Reduced Doses

Aspirin doses should be reduced, but not necessarily eliminated, for children, underweight adults and some persons with unusual sensitivity to aspirin.

Drug doses are generally related to body weight. Since children weigh less than adults, a given aspirin dose has a greater effect on them. The same goes for grossly underweight adults. But children are especially vulnerable to aspirin side effects because their drug-handling systems are less well developed and easier to upset.

As a general rule, children under the age of two, or those taking medication, should never be given aspirin without consulting a physician.

An FDA advisory panel recommends children's aspirin tablets be used until age twelve. These tablets typically contain 75 to 80 milligrams of aspirin, about one-fourth the adult dose of 325 milligrams. For healthy children of normal weight, the panel recommends these doses of 80 milligram tablets, every four hours:

Age	Tablets
2–4	two
4–6	three
6–8	four
8–10	five
10–12	six

Above age twelve, a young person can be given two adult-size tablets. If children's aspirin is unavailable, one adult tablet may be given to a child above the age of six.

A person's sensitivity to a given dose of aspirin can vary depending on a number of conditions, including diet, use of vitamins and non-prescription drugs and general health. In addition, each person has a unique reaction to drugs that depends on their genetic makeup. Any of these factors can result in occasional side effects

23

at dose levels that are normally well tolerated; in such cases, reduce aspirin doses.

How to Buy Aspirin

The selection of an aspirin brand vexes many people, although it should not. All commercially available brands of aspirin, or aspirin compounds, provide roughly equal relief. Compounds and pure aspirin vary only slightly in effectiveness and side effects. Different brands of pure aspirin also vary only slightly.

These slight differences are not significant to the vast majority of those who take aspirin for an occasional headache. But arthritics sometimes take twenty tablets a day, and about 2 percent of the population regularly gets heartburn from taking aspirin: for these people, and some others, even a slight difference in effectiveness or side effects may loom large indeed.

How can such differences be determined? Price is not a reliable barometer of quality among aspirin and aspirin compound brands. As of early 1977, the price of 100 tablets varied between 14 cents and $1.43. Tests by the Good Housekeeping Institute found Bayer, at $1.39, consistently pure; while some brands didn't fare as well, one 14-cent house brand tested by the Institute received a rating similar to that of Bayer. The maximum price difference of $1.25 is, however, slight for the casual aspirin user. Only those who take a great deal of aspirin are likely to find it worth their time and trouble to test various brands (testing methods are described later in this chapter) and select the best.

Buying Pure Aspirin

The similarities between brands of pure aspirin are greater than their differences. One study, reported in the *Journal of the American Medical Association*, found no pain-relieving difference between Bayer and St. Joseph's, two nationally advertised brands of aspirin.

The Arthritis Foundation, concerned about aspirin in view of the fact that half of all aspirin is taken by arthritics, found brand names make no difference. "Unadvertised brands of aspirin are just as effective as 'name' brands and cost far less. Aspirin is aspirin, regardless of the commercial name attached to it," according to the foundation.

Consumers Union reports that there is no reason not to buy the least expensive aspirin available, since "aspirin is aspirin. The only practical difference for most people is price."

On the other hand, aspirin manufacturers contend that manufacturing technique does make a difference in effectiveness. A pharmaceutical-industry publication cites research done in a Boston hospital that concluded: "It is apparent from our experience that some products are more carefully manufactured and better tolerated by patients." The researchers attributed the different tolerances to variation in the rate of tablet disintegration, which in turn affects the rate of stomach upset.

Stomach upset and absorption speed do vary between aspirin brands, according to the American Pharmaceutical Association's *Handbook*, which noted, "The statement frequently heard that all aspirin products are alike is naive and in complete contradiction to the voluminous mass of published data on the subject."

Indeed, there are differences between brands of aspirin. The question remains whether these differences are significant. Except at the extremes of manufacturing quality, the answer is no. For most people, most brands of pure aspirin will produce similar results.

Tests to Perform

Different manufacturers make various brands of aspirin in a variety of ways. Some home tests can determine whether an aspirin brand meets standards; other standards cannot be tested at home, but can be checked indirectly.

The first test is to read the label; the initials USP are the manufacturer's assurance it has met minimum requirements of the U.S. Pharmacopoeia, an independent non-profit agency that compiles standards. Even when the initials are not present, most products that claim to be aspirin meet these standards. They are only minimum requirements; some manufacturers meet them, some exceed the standards.

One USP standard you can test directly at home is disintegration time. Researchers believe disintegration time is related to stomach upset; the faster aspirin disintegrates, the less stomach distress. The USP standard is five minutes; the Good Housekeeping Institute says a tablet in a warm saucer of water should disintegrate when touched after two minutes. Bayer, for example, allows thirty seconds. In judging disintegration time, faster is better: five minutes is the longest time allowable, but two minutes is a more reasonable standard.

USP standard aspirin should be pure white and odorless, two characteristics that can be tested at home. If aspirin is gray or smells like vinegar, it is less effective and causes more side effects. Discoloration or a vinegar smell are caused by age or moisture in the bottle; aspirin deteriorated by either of these factors should be thrown away. Since aspirin is often kept in steamy bathrooms, the deterioration problem is not uncommon but can be reduced by immediately removing the cotton in the top when the bottle is opened and resealing the cap tightly after each use.

Other attributes of high-quality aspirin cannot be tested directly at home, such as purity and quality control during the manufacturing process. Incorrect tablet count and broken tablets are two frequent indicators of careless manufacturing. Aspects of the manufacturing process that cannot be checked at home may be presumed correct if the count is correct and the tablets are whole.

The largest study of variations in aspirin brand characteristics was completed in 1971 by Sterling Drug Inc., maker of Bayer aspirin. Sterling compared 221 brands of aspirin during a period of four years. It found 5 percent of the samples did not meet USP standards for aspirin content per tablet or dissolving time. Sterling found 84 percent of the brands were short one or more tablets in one or more samples. The company found 45 percent of the bottles in the study had a vinegar smell.

Buying Aspirin Compounds

Available data does not prove either tolerance or effectiveness of aspirin is increased by adding ingredients, despite loud proclamations to the contrary by several manufacturers. The question of differences between plain aspirin and aspirin compounds is shrouded in controversy, but presently available evidence indicates such differences are slight, if they exist at all.

To some aspirin-takers, however, even a slight difference can be important, so the more widely advertised combination products will be described.

On a general note, the APHA *Handbook* stated, "These combinations, for the most part, are of greater economic significance to the manufacturer than increased therapeutic benefit to the patient." Most researchers believe combination products are usually no more effective than the single strongest drug in the combination. In fact, they find effectiveness is not additive, but that side effects are.

Before discussing specific brands, it should be noted that some compounds could be changed by the 1980s. The Food and Drug Administration reviews non-prescription drugs for safety and effectiveness. To reduce side effects, an FDA advisory panel has suggested that no single product should contain more than two pain-killing ingredients. APC and Excedrin, for example, each contain three pain-killers, as do other products that are less widely known. The FDA panel's suggestions presently lack the force of law and may take years to implement, if accepted by the FDA.

Bufferin, and house brands of similar composition, are aspirin compounds that claim to reduce stomach distress by providing a small amount of antacid with their aspirin. The amount of antacid is insufficient to neutralize the acid in the aspirin, but is believed

27

by some physicians to be sufficient to decrease stomach irritation and slightly increase the speed of absorption into the bloodstream. Others suggest the decreased irritation may result from the power of suggestion: if one firmly believes a pill will reduce stomach up-set, it may well happen.

Dr. William T. Beaver of the Sloan-Kettering Cancer Institute in New York found stomach upset from aspirin was rare. He wrote, "Many patients who maintain they cannot tolerate aspirin do so quite well if the drug is given on a blind basis, or disguised as a more elegant preparation."

Buffered aspirin has not proven its ability to reduce upset or increase absorption speed. The AMA *Drug Evaluations* stated buf-fered aspirin has not been "conclusively shown to be either faster or gentler."

Alka-Seltzer, another compound of antacid and aspirin, does contain enough antacid to neutralize the acid in the aspirin, which is its active pain-killing ingredient. This brand poses other prob-lems, however. Persons on low-salt diets should avoid it because of its high sodium content. Alka-Seltzer takes effect slightly faster than regular aspirin, but its effect may not last as long. And, if used frequently, Alka-Seltzer builds up a chemical reaction in the intes-tines that slows absorption. Alka-Seltzer causes less stomach bleed-ing than aspirin, because it is already dissolved when swallowed and because its acid is neutralized. But stomach bleeding after tak-ing aspirin is trivial in most persons. Alka-Seltzer is some twenty times more expensive than everyday aspirin, so it may not seem worth the investment.

Excedrin and Anacin combine caffeine with aspirin, claiming it is a pain-reliever, a thesis rejected by the FDA advisory panel on OTC pain-killers. Drug companies claim that, in some migraine headaches, caffeine reduces pain by decreasing blood vessel con-striction. But a cup of coffee provides twice the caffeine of Exced-rin and four times that of Anacin. The AMA *Drug Evaluations* con-cludes caffeine has no pain-killing effect in small doses and does not add to the effects of aspirin.

In a class by itself as an additive to aspirin compounds is

phenacetin, found in APC tablets, Bromo-Seltzer, and Empirin compound as of early 1977. In much of Europe, phenacetin is available only by prescription and it has already been banned from aspirin compounds in Canada. The FDA advisory panel has recommended phenacetin be taken off the market as an OTC drug and made a prescription drug. Its use was once widespread, but phenacetin has been associated with permanent kidney damage at high, sustained doses. All products containing the drug already carry an FDA-required warning: "may damage the kidneys when used in large amounts for a long period of time." Unless the FDA advisory panel is overruled, phenacetin will soon disappear from non-prescription pain-relief products.

Aspirin Substitutes

Take aspirin for minor pain unless there are clear reasons to avoid the drug. Available substitutes are often more expensive, or less effective.

If an individual should avoid aspirin, the best available non-prescription substitute is acetaminophen, sold "straight" under such names as Datril and Tylenol or in compounds, such as Bromo-Seltzer, among other brands.

Acetaminophen, often more expensive than aspirin, reduces pain and fewer but not inflammation, and has no effect on the clotting system. Thus, it is less effective in treating inflammation-based pain, such as arthritis, and could not have the same effect in reducing heart-attack risk as aspirin is believed to have.

The relative safety of acetaminophen and aspirin has been cast into doubt. The FDA advisory panel recommends warning labels on acetaminophen that point out the danger of liver damage in overdose, a warning not required on aspirin. In addition, the panel said some acetaminophen advertising gives the impression that it is much safer than aspirin, a claim the panel found baseless.

A massive aspirin overdose leads to death more rapidly than an acetaminophen overdose, but aspirin poisoning is easier to recognize and treat at the onset. Because of its symptoms, ringing ears and nausea, an aspirin overdose may be recognized immediately, while an acetaminophen overdose may delay its major symptom, yellowing skin due to liver failure, for two or three days. Then it may be too late for treatment.

Ingredients of Aspirin Compounds

An FDA advisory panel has found six ingredients safe and effective for pain and fever relief: acetaminophen, aspirin, calcium carbaspirin, choline salicylate, magnesium salicylate, and sodium salicylate. All but the first are chemical relatives of aspirin, and all but the first two are used only rarely.

As compiled by the American Pharmaceutical Association, here are the ingredients of the most popular pain-relief products:

Alka-Seltzer: 324 milligrams (mg) aspirin, 1.9 grams (g) sodium bicarbonate, 1.0 g citric acid.

Anacin: 400 mg aspirin, 32.5 mg caffeine.

ASA Compound (also, most drugs called APC): 227 mg aspirin, 160 mg phenacetin, 32.5 mg caffeine.

Bayer Aspirin: 324 mg aspirin.

Bayer Children's Aspirin: 81 mg aspirin.

Bromo-Seltzer: (per capful) 130 mg phenacetin, 325 mg acetaminophen, 32.5 mg caffeine, 2.8 g of sodium bicarbonate and citric acid, in sodium citrate form.

Bufferin: 324 mg aspirin, 97.2 mg magnesium carbonate, 48.6 mg aluminum glycinate (antacids).

Empirin Compound: 227 mg aspirin, 162 mg. phenacetin, 32 mg caffeine.

Excedrin: 194.4 mg aspirin, 129.6 mg salicylamide (pain killer from the aspirin chemical family), 97 mg acetaminophen, 64.8 mg caffeine.

St. Joseph Aspirin: 325 mg aspirin.

St. Joseph Aspirin for Children: 81 mg aspirin.

Tylenol: 325 mg acetaminophen.

Groundless Myths

Some members of the public believe continuing doses of aspirin will result in a tolerance to the drug, requiring larger and larger doses to achieve the same effect. It is possible to develop a tolerance for some drugs, but aspirin is not one of them.

Drs. Martin Gross and Leon Goldberg of Yale Medical School examined fifty years of aspirin research and concluded the drug leads neither to tolerance nor addiction. They found no case in which an individual required increased doses to achieve the same effect, and added, "It [aspirin] is habit-forming only to the extent that frequent use of any substance which gives relief, real or imagined, from pain, is a habit."

Another large segment of the population is concerned about taking aspirin in the general context of a society in which too many drugs are taken and the specific context of introducing artificial substances into the body.

Whether or not aspirin is "artificial" is a point for semantic quibbling. It is synthetic, manufactured from coal and oil; but as described in Chapter 3, aspirin's discovery was the result of efforts to isolate the effective pain killer in willow bark, used to kill pain for thousands of years when supply never came close to demand. Modern chemistry has merely made a stronger relative of this compound more readily available through synthesis of what is, basically, a natural substance.

Dr. James S. Schoenberger heads a major aspirin study, described in Chapter 7. He was asked about the fear that drugs in general are too popular:

> Every drug carries with it some risk. On the other hand, to say to someone who has pneumonia, "We are not going to give you penicillin" is foolhardy. So I don't think you can make a general statement we have gone too far with the use of drugs. When you look at the miracle which happened with tuberculosis or poliomyelitis or pneumonia, it makes that an academic, sterile comment. A modern American physician has a host of good drugs

which should be used and used properly. What you are going to get into otherwise is some mystical ways with less scientific validity than drugs.

Conclusion

Easily maligned but even more easily defended, aspirin could readily be called the easy medicine. It is also easy to take properly, easy to buy, and easy to know when to avoid (if sometimes difficult to avoid). However, aspirin was not easy to find; more than a century elapsed between the first tentative chemical steps toward isolation of the drug and its final triumphant emergence from a German pharmaceutical laboratory.

3

The History of Aspirin

The story of aspirin extends from the taking of certain herbs in the earliest days of recorded history to today's $700 million dollar a year industry, upon which the sun never sets. It is a story of misplaced discoveries, missed opportunities and sometimes misadvised expenditures. In the end, aspirin's manufacture today in a pure, consistent, inexpensive form is a triumph of pharmaceutical technology.

Early pain relievers were no such pharmaceutical triumph. Archeological evidence indicates that primitive peoples used all kinds of roots, herbs, and natural substances for medicinal purposes. Most of these apparently achieved their effect through faith in their ability to heal. Modern medicine has often been unable to find a rational chemical explanation for most herbs' supposed effects. But some of these substances worked because they contained chemicals that actually were physiologically effective. These herbals led early medical practitioners to their first important pharmaceutical discoveries: opium for pain, digitalis for heart problems, and quinine for malaria.

The search for a safe, non-addictive pain reliever has occupied medical practitioners since antiquity. Hippocrates, the father of

33

modern medicine, was the first to propose an aspirin-like substance for the reduction of pain. He recorded the details of medical practice 2,300 years ago, and originated the physician's rule, "Be useful, or at least do no harm."

Hippocrates found willow leaves were a pain reliever that met his standard and recommended they be given to women during childbirth, since chewing on them seemed to reduce pain. A good part of the effect came from "biting the bullet," that is, distraction from the source of pain. But another portion of the relief resulted from the naturally occuring form of aspirin—salicin—present in the leaves.

The next recorded description of willow leaves taken to reduce pain is that of Dioscorides, a Greek surgeon in the Roman military service. In 75 A.D. he listed the medicinal herbs known at the time, including willow leaf, beaten and drunk with pepper and wine to "help such as are troubled with stomach pains." He also found willow leaves useful in the treatment of gout—perhaps because salicin, like aspirin, can both relieve the pain and control the cause of gout (see Chapter 5).

A Roman encyclopedia writer, Pliny the Elder, mentioned the willow leaf as a pain killer, as did Galen. The latter, a Greek-educated Roman physician, wrote a thirty-volume encyclopedia near the end of the second century A.D. In it, he listed pain, fever, and inflammation as symptoms controlled by willow leaves; the same symptoms controlled by aspirin today.

After the second century, there was no further progress in understanding the source of the willow's palliative power until the nineteenth century.

Use of various herbs for medicinal purposes, of course, continued during the intervening 1,700 years, but without clear understanding of how they worked, or why. Willow leaves and roots were favored in Europe to reduce the pain of earache and gout. In America, the Indians drank a liquid that included juice from willow-tree bark to reduce fever. The early Pennsylvania Germans, possibly on the advice of the Indians, extracted medicine from a plant called Shepherd's Purse, which contains salicin, to combat fevers caused by dysentery.

After a gap of 1,300 or so years, written notation of willow leaves as pain relievers appeared again during the 1500s, as Dodoens, court physician of Austro-Hungarian Emperor Maximillian II, wrote that leaves boiled in wine would "appease the pain of the sinews and does restore again their strength."

First Chemical Forms

With the rise of the scientific method and its recognition of cause and effect relationships, the pace of medical and pharmaceutical developments began to quicken in the eighteenth century.

Fever reduction was the first medical task to benefit from the new approach, which led to the discovery of salicin as a by-product of the search for quinine. In England, quinine was first called "Peruvian Bark" after the region where it was discovered by Spanish explorers, who found that chewing on it reduced fevers, or "ague." The bark, also known as cinchona, was first believed to reduce all fevers and thought to fail only when doses were insufficient. It was nearly a century before "ague" was discovered to be a number of diseases, only one of which, malaria, could be controlled by cinchona or quinine, the component of the bark that killed malarial parasites.

In 1757, however, a shortage of Peruvian Bark in Great Britain led Reverend Edmund Stone of Chipping-Norton, Oxfordshire, to search for a readily available substitute to allay fevers. There is no record of his search process, but chances are he overheard village women discuss the properties of willow bark.

Stone, who also practiced medicine, in the custom of his time, was intrigued; he had tasted bitter cinchona and knew it was a dried, powered preparation of bark. He then tried dried, powdered willow bark and discovered it had a similar taste.

In his own view, the reverend's discovery was not by luck, since he searched for a substitute in a swampy area because of his belief in the "doctrine of signatures," a popular theory of his time. In Stone's words: "As this tree [willow] delights in a moist or wet soil, where agues [fevers] chiefly abound, the general maxim that many natural maladies carry their cures with them, or that their remedies lie not far from their causes, was so very apposite to this particular case that he could not help applying it [Stone referred to himself in the third person]." In short, malaria and other diseases characterized by fever were more common in swampy areas, so Stone looked there for a cure.

For whatever reason, Stone tried willow bark as a fever reducer, taking the first step on the road to discovery of aspirin. He sent word of his discovery to the Royal Society of London, which published it in the journal *Philosophical Transactions* in April, 1763. For five years, Stone said, he had prescribed willow-bark powder to reduce fever. Fifty persons had used it and only a few stubborn fevers had continued; even these were reduced slightly, Stone wrote. The patients took the powder with beer, tea, or water and were not "prepared" as patients customarily were then, by bleeding or vomiting. Stone reported with glee that dried, powdered willow bark was "a safe medicine for he never could perceive the least ill effect from it." Although he did not say how he arrived at the figure, Stone did report that he gave his patients the powder once every four hours.

Laboratory Work Begins

As the nineteenth century began, medical science moved from fields and meadows and informal pharmacies (run by alchemists, primarily) into the newly formed chemical laboratories of Europe. Early chemists worked first to extract the active ingredients of already proven herbal cures. By the middle of the century, chemistry developed to the point that synthesis of these ingredients (their creation from non-plant substances) would be possible.

Aspirin and many other drugs would emerge from this laboratory revolution, which contributed substantially to the increase of European and North American life spans, from forty-five years to seventy years.

One of the major products of the laboratory revolution was the pain-reliever aspirin, discovered incidentally during the scientific

36

search for drugs that would reduce fever. Throughout the nineteenth century, physicians believed fever was a cause of illness. It was not until the twentieth century that they learned it was a symptom, indicating the body's efforts to fight disease, and not a cause. Cinchona shortages and concern about fever as a disease cause set pharmaceutical labs searching for pure anti-pyretic, or fever-reducing, substances.

The first success in the search for chemically pure fever reducers, another step on the road to aspirin, came in Italy. There, in 1826, two chemists extracted small amounts of salicin, the active anti-pyretic ingredient of willow bark, during a project believed inspired by Stone's pioneering work.

In 1832, a Swiss pharmacist found meadowsweet, one of the shrubs of the spirea family, yielded a much greater percentage of salicin than willow bark. He sent this salicin to German chemist Karl Jakob Löwig. In one of his experiments with the salicin, Löwig created salicylic acid (SA), which he called "Spirsäure," after the plant family from which it was derived. His name for the acid would later become part of the word "aspirin."

Salicylic acid (SA) is the substance from which aspirin is made today. But before it could be experimented upon by large numbers of chemists, it had to be readily available: as long as SA was derived from plants, this was hardly possible. Thus, the 1860 announcement of a practical method of SA synthesis by Herman Kolbe and his collaborator was an important step toward aspirin's discovery.

In Strasbourg, Charles Frederic von Gerhardt conducted experiments on plant-derived SA and unwittingly discovered aspirin. Starting in 1853, he combined SA with various other substances, including a chemical salt that yielded acetylsalicylic acid, ASA or aspirin. Von Gerhardt made the first recorded discovery of the substance, but did not discover its effects. His work came too soon for him to envision ASA as a drug—it was two decades before medical use of SA became common. Thus, ASA became a laboratory curiosity that spent forty years in the back pages of books listing apparently useless chemical combinations. $C_9H_8O_4$ had not yet found its moment.

Salicylic acid, on the other hand, was emerging as a useful

substance for the preservation of meat and milk. The growth of its importance, which would lead to discovery of ASA's effects, began with seemingly unrelated events in Scotland.

Joseph Lister, a surgeon working in Glasgow, had discovered the existence of infection and found that washing a patient's skin with carbolic acid prior to an operation achieved disinfection.

A physician who knew both Kolbe and Lister theorized that carbolic acid, which killed germs on the skin, might also kill them internally. But there was a problem: carbolic acid was poisonous when taken orally. The man assumed carbolic acid would not be poisonous if ingested in another form and broken down within the body. He asked Kolbe if there was such a compound.

The question reminded Kolbe of his experiments that led to SA synthesis. One of the problems he had faced in synthesizing SA was its tendency to break down into component parts, one of which was carbolic acid. Kolbe performed new experiments on salicylic acid when this "internal disinfectant" was proposed. He tested SA on animals, then on humans, to determine its safety. Finally, in 1874, Kolbe wrote a paper describing the use of SA as an internal disinfectant.

SA was the first synthetic drug to play a major role in medicine and, as such, generated unusual excitement when it was introduced. Many doctors rushed samples of the acid from laboratories to patients, without knowing how it worked or which diseases it would affect.

After several years of testing, physicians concluded salicylic acid would not cure diseases, as they had hoped it would, but that it reduced fever, then thought to be a disease cause. And some doctors noted an incidental effect: SA reduced pain and inflammation.

Also in 1874, the usefulness of the aspirin chemical family was praised in another important medical paper. Scottish physician T. J. MacLagan reported on his work with salicin:

> I had at the time under my care a well-marked case of the disease [rheumatism] which was being treated with alkalies but was not improving. I determined to give him sali-

cin; but before doing so, took myself first five, then 10, then 30 grains [a quantity equal in bulk, but not effectiveness, to 6 aspirin tablets] without experiencing the least inconvenience or discomfort. Satisfied as to the safety of its administration, I gave to the patient refered to 12 grains every three hours. The results exceeded my most sanguine expectations . . . . When given at the commencement of the attack [of pain], it seems sometimes to arrest the course of the malady.

The Discovery of Aspirin

Dr. MacLagan may well have found salicin free of side effects in the doses he used; the drug's more powerful and useful cousin, SA, was less benign. It was an acid that burned the mouth and throat as it was swallowed. Upon receiving salicylic acid, a person's stomach felt like it was "crawling with ants." While SA lowered fever and relieved pain, it was administered in an alcoholic liquid that tasted sickeningly sweet and often caused vomiting and unconsciousness.

Despite its side effects, the widespread use of SA launched the first major wave of drug discoveries in Europe. It was called the anti-pyretic wave, because the drugs sought were intended primarily to reduce fever, These drugs were usually discovered by German chemical firms, because they had Europe's only large-scale laboratories. The drugs were petroleum-based because of the German firms' experience in the petrochemical textile dye business.

As part of the wave, in 1876, sodium salicylate was synthesized, followed in 1885 by phenyl salicylate. These two substances were created by "taming" SA—attempting to reduce its side effects by adding other substances to the basic acid. Other techniques led to discovery of other substances, but "taming" brought forth most of the useful pain and fever reducers; however, they still tasted bad and burned the mouth, stomach, and throat.

The only salicylic acid derivative still commonly used today is aspirin, or ASA. Its properties were discovered in the phar-macological laboratory of "Farberfabriken vorm. Friedr. Bayer & Co.," at Elberfeld, Germany, which in 1925 became a division of the giant I.G. Farbenindustrie drug and dye trust. The successor firm is known today as Farbenfabriken Bayer GmbH, or Bayer AG, of Leverkusen, West Germany.

In 1893, Felix Hoffman worked for Bayer as a research chem-ist. One of his assignments was to look for a new and better yellow dye. But the popularity of SA, despite irritating side effects, led Bayer to a corporate goal: find a less irritating anti-pyretic drug. Hoffman was one of the chemists put to work on the new as-signment.

Hoffman had company orders for motivation, but he also had something extra: the intense pain his father suffered. The elder Hoffman was cruelly wracked with rheumatoid arthritis. He could no longer tolerate any of the already-discovered salicylate sub-stances, but his need for relief was intense. He implored his son to search for a drug he could take without nausea.

Spurred by his double motivation, Hoffman conducted a thor-ough search of published papers on SA and its derivatives. In one of them, he found a description of the chemical makeup of ASA as written by the man who first synthesized it, von Gerhardt.

Hoffman did more than look up ASA in a book; the von Ger-hardt method of synthesis was complicated, impractical for mass manufacture. Hoffman simplified the process, producing a bitter, silky white powder. He tested it on himself, without side effects, then gave it to his father, who found pain relief without side effects for the first time in years. ASA was as effective as the plain salicylic acid, but had virtually none of SA's side effects.

In 1897, Hoffman took his seemingly well-tested discovery to his immediate supervisor, who was so impressed he immediately presented ASA to Dr. Heinrich Dreser, head of the Bayer phar-macology section. Dreser was initially rather skeptical, referring to the newly isolated drug as a "direct heart poison" and a useless product. But company history indicates that after further tests, he came to recognize the value of aspirin.

Dreser's support was important if aspirin was to gain widespread acceptance quickly. He was widely known among European chemists, having introduced heroin as a substitute for morphine in the 1880's. His personal backing would lend nearly instant respectability to a new drug.

Dreser, in an 1899 medical journal paper, described one experiment he conducted that helped change his mind about the drug.

> The local reaction of the salicylic acid on the stomach is irritation. In order to compare aspirin with salicylic acid in this respect, I have found the transparent swimming fin of a small fish very suitable.
>
> [I would] wrap up the fish in a narrow, wet linen bandage and then respire it artifically by installing a rubber hose in its mouth and a syphon to let fresh water trickle over its gills. Then I simply let the stabilizer fin hang freely over a little tray and dipped it in a small dish containing the solutions I was comparing.
>
> [One dish contained aspirin, the other SA, both dissolved in water.] A difference was noticeable in less than one minute. The treated fins became distinctly more opaque in SA than in ASA.

Dreser speculated that the fins had the same sensitivity to irritation as the human stomach, and proved with tests on himself, that this was true: ASA, or aspirin, caused less stomach upset than SA.

Once Dreser was won over to support the new drug, he became personally involved in its promotion, shipping samples to German physicians. Then, in 1899, he published his own description of the discovery process, in the same issue as the glowing clinical reports of two doctors who had found aspirin effective for relief of pain and fever.

Prior to publication, Hoffman and Dreser realized that acetylsalicylic acid needed to have a trade name. The scientific name was hard to pronounce and hard to remember. Besides, a generic name like ASA could not be patented; only specific trade names could be protected from commercial competitors.

Hoffman wanted to call the drug a-salacin, or a-salicylic, simply abbreviating the "acetyl" part of the name. Dreser did not think that was simple enough. He recalled Löwig's name for SA, "Spirsäure." Dreser took Hoffman's idea, abbreviating the acetyl to "a," then added "spir" for "Spirsäure" and "in" as a suffix.

The result was "aspirin," spelled the same in German and English, easy to pronouce and easy to remember. The cleverness of the name may have contributed to aspirin's rapid acceptance at the turn of the century, a time when the attention of doctors was diverted by a bewildering array of new drug introductions.

The difficulty of keeping all the new drugs straight was described in a paper that outlined early aspirin tests:

> [New drugs] are thrown on the market almost every day, and one needs a marvelous memory if one wants to remember all the new names. Many pop up, are praised and recommended by a few authors and especially by the manufacturers, and after a short time, one hears no more of them.

Aspirin Comes to America

The powder that Dreser described as having a "pleasant sharp taste" was introduced into the United States in 1900. No tests of its effectiveness or safety were required; the manufacturer simply made it available to pharmacists and informed doctors of its utility. The only brake on widespread aspirin-taking was aspirin's clumsy form; as a powder, it had to be placed in envelopes and capsules by pharmacists, making it expensive and inconvenient.

As Bayer AG learned to make aspirin in tablet form, shortly before World War I, the price became so low that "no obstacle stands in the way" of its universal use, the company said. In fact, however, early tablets were crude and tended to cause more stomach upset than the powdered form. For several years, both forms were marketed. Then, in 1915, the tablet-making process was markedly improved. Since 1915, aspirin has been available over the counter, without pharmacist intervention for weighing and packing.

Prior to 1917, only the Bayer Company of New York, then a subsidiary of Bayer AG, made aspirin in the United States. But in that year, the American patent on the substance expired, and a large American chemical firm, the Monsanto Co. of St. Louis, began making aspirin. In 1921 the Bayer Company lost a court suit to protect the name and the compound, both of which then permanently entered the public domain.

During World War I the Bayer Company had passed out of German hands, when the U.S. Government seized the company's stock as being held by enemy aliens. The Alien Property Custodian in 1918 offered the stock at a public auction in which many American firms took part. Sterling Products, now Sterling Drug Inc., made the high bid, and thus acquired the company's assets, including the rights to the Bayer name. As a result, the United States, Canada, and parts of the Carribean are the only parts of the world in which Bayer AG is not the sole manufacturer of aspirin, under the Bayer name.

Aspirin Manufacturing

Sterling Drug Inc., Monsanto Co., Dow Chemical, Tenneco Chemicals Inc., Miles Laboratories, and Norwich Co. are the six major U.S. chemical firms that make aspirin. The firms that sell Anacin, Bufferin, Excedrin, St. Joseph's, and many other brands of aspirin or aspirin compounds do not make their own aspirin; they buy it from these firms, in bulk. ASA is received either as a powder to mix with other ingredients, or as a tablet ready to be sold under a trade name. Sterling (Bayer), Miles (Alka-Seltzer), and Norwich (Norwich Aspirin) manufacture their own aspirin from salicylic acid they buy.

The manufacturing process starts with coal tar or petroleum.

From a light petroleum fraction salicylic acid is formed. The SA must be "tamed" by the addition of an acetyl group of atoms, making it into acetylsalicylic acid, or aspirin. There are several different methods for accomplishing acetylation. But they all have one thing in common; the processes are completely mechanical. ASA is never touched by human hands, until the bottle is opened by the consumer.

The basic steps of the Sterling method are public. The process generally takes five days and is usually started each Monday to conclude by Friday. The SA is delivered to a New Jersey plant in fiber drums, then pumped into stainless-steel tanks that hold 550 gallons, or about 1,800 pounds, of chemicals used in aspirin-making. The tanks are heated to near boiling, then agitated continuously, like a washing machine in the spin cycle, at up to eighty revolutions per minute. The SA reacts with other chemicals in the tank, and turns into ASA and by-products, the ASA drops to the bottom of the tank, where it is washed with a non-aqueous solvent, filtered, and dried. Sterling does not use water in its "non-aqueous" process, because water reacts with aspirin to form acetic acid (vinegar) when exposed to air. Other firms avoid vinegar by drying their aspirin or by separating out the acetic acid.

The proportions of aspirin, unreacted by-products, acetic acid, and unchanged salicylic acid vary among the different processes. Because these impurities can reduce effectiveness, speed deterioration or increase side effects, the choice of manufacturing method is important.

After the manufacturing stage, the differences between manufacturers are few. To make aspirin tablets, the glistening, white crystalline powder is filtered and dried after acetylation. It is then mixed with fillers, such as corn starch or talc (a refined form of the substance used to make talcum powder). Sterling makes Bayer with an 80 percent aspirin–20 percent cornstarch mixture; other firms mix aspirin 80-20 or 90-10 with starch, starch and talc, or other neutral substances.

In the Sterling process, aspirin and tablet-making filler are mixed in one-ton batches. The two substances are very thoroughly mixed, to avoid an imbalance in the filler-aspirin ratio of any single tablet. Large stamping presses then compress the powdered aspirin, under fifteen tons of pressure, into "slugs" the weight of sixteen tablets.

These slugs are then ground until they are only small particles, differing from the original powder in that each particle is a consistently sized grouping of many aspirin crystals mixed with filler. These particles are fed into a tablet press, which produces 3,000 tablets a minute under two and a half tons of pressure.

The tablets are then run by conveyor belt into a vertical drop shoot divided into five sections. Operated by weight, each section, one after the other, drops 20 tablets at a time into a 100-tablet container (different counts are used for different containers).

Machines then insert cotton into the bottle, attach labels, affix the child-resistant cap and place the container in a carton.

Aspirin's Image

Like most over-the-counter drugs, aspirin is heavily advertised. One aspirin-containing product, Anacin, spends more than $26 million a year on advertising.

The effect of advertising on product cost (and perhaps sales) can be examined by a comparison of 1975 advertising costs and wholesale values compiled by the author:

Brand	Advertising (millions)	Value of sales (millions)	Advertising as a percentage
Anacin	$26.2	$75	35%
Bufferin	14.5	55	26%
Excedrin	11.7	54	22%
Bayer	10.8	68	16%

Two comments about the table are in order. First, only one aspirin, Bayer, makes the top four list. The other products are combinations; as noted before, extra ingredients are more important for improving profits than for improving relief. Second, advertising expense order is the same as wholesale value order, except for Bayer. That exception may be the result of the product's unusual brand name familiarity and decades-long head start.

Today's advertising for aspirin deals with the range of problems (real and imagined) associated with aspirin in the public mind; stomach upset, strength, and speed of relief. In 1976, most advertising was handled in a manner different from that of the 50s and 60s, when little a's chased little b's through plastic stomachs. Some television critics claimed animated hammers pounding on little anvils inside people's heads on television, or announcers shouting "fast, fast, fast" boosted pain-reliever sales partly by causing headaches themselves.

Today, advertisements for aspirin are quieter, but with a marked tendency to ignore uncomfortable facts: Anacin never mentions that aspirin is the "pain reliever doctors specify most;" Bufferin seldom discusses studies that disprove its claim to be "faster and gentler to the stomach;" and TV star spokesmen for Excedrin do not tout the FDA panel suggestion that products with one or two pain relievers have fewer side effects than those with three, such as Excedrin.

Advertising was simpler during aspirin's early years, perhaps because there was less competition. A 1918 advertisement for Bayer says nothing about speed, strength, or stomach upset. It merely informs the reader of Bayer's purity and the location of the manufacturing plant, and displays a picture of this solid edifice, with smokestacks puffing prosperously.

Any product as heavily used and advertised as aspirin makes frequent appearances in the popular culture. The drug appears in comic strips, plays, and movies. A Connecticut firm that claims to relieve the "headaches" of workman's compensation refers to itself as "The Big Aspirin" in an advertisement. "Take two and call me in the morning" is a cartoon punchline, time and again. In television situation comedies, reaching for or taking aspirin is as sure a sign of impending trouble as the audience saying "uh-oh."

The great and seemingly untraceable myth about aspirin is that if you drop it into a glass of Coke and drink it, you will get high. Physiologically, there is no basis for this persistent folklore. However, at least since the 1920s, several generations of giggling teenagers have gathered in party rooms from coast to coast to drink the concoction. For them, it seems to work.

The Coca-Cola Company's public-relations people in Atlanta are periodically asked about the combination of Coke and aspirin. A company spokesman says no one knows where the myth got started and that all inquiries are answered firmly in the negative. The most likely explanation of the myth is the power of suggestion; if you want to get high on Coke and aspirin, you might very well do so.

If Aspirin Were New Today

The only barriers to rapid introduction of new drugs at the turn of the century, when aspirin was introduced, were marketing and manufacturing. There was no government protection; unless side effects were frequent and fatal they were seldom discussed.

Would the Food and Drug Administration disapprove of aspirin if it were introduced today? "I don't know whether we can make that bold statement," an FDA spokesman said. Stomach problems and the still-developing understanding of how the drug works might give the agency pause, but "If all we knew about aspirin were now presented to the FDA it would be approved," probably as a prescription drug, as are most new drugs, he said. If years of use indicated the possibility of safe self-administration, it might later become over-the-counter. Aspirin's easy OTC availability today is a quirk of history.

A detailed explanation of how aspirin works would aid this hypothetical conversion from prescription to non-prescription. After more than seventy years, medical scientists have developed such an explanation in the last few years; it is presented in the next chapter.

4

What It Does; How It Works

Aspirin relieves the common symptoms of pain, fever, and inflammation quickly, effectively and with few side effects. Aspirin's relatives have relieved these symptoms for centuries, starting with the Roman use of willow bark to kill pain. Shortly after aspirin itself was marketed in 1899, medical studies proved it effective for these three symptoms; it has remained the most effective drug for pain, fever, and inflammation in the intervening seventy-eight years.

Yet until the 1970s, no one was certain how aspirin worked inside the human system. It was not until the mid-1970s that a majority of medical researchers would agree they knew a good deal about how aspirin achieved its effects. Today, with this new understanding, they are exploring aspirin's possibilities in cancer therapy, in the control of reproduction and in wide-scale reduction of heart-attack and stroke risk.

Pain

Pain has been humanity's malign companion since the process of evolution developed a nervous system capable of registering it. Aristotle, thousands of years before Christ, called it a "passion of the soul." Another ancient Greek physician, Antiphanes, wrote, "All pain's one malady, with many names." He might well have added the most popular: "Unwanted."

During the middle ages, theories about pain became more focused; it was viewed as punishment for sin, or as a test by God of a person's fortitude. Buddha, for example, said, "Pain is the outcome of sin." If philosophers have had trouble being lucid about pain, perhaps Shakespeare had an explanation: "There was never yet philosopher that could endure toothache patiently." (Leonato, *Much Ado About Nothing*, Act V, Sc. I, 1. 36)

The American poet William Cullen Bryant mused about pain in verse:

> They talk of short-lived pleasures, be it so;
> Pain dies as quickly, and lets her sweaty prisoner go;
> The fiercest agonies have the shortest reign.

Physicians have had little better luck in their efforts to describe pain; their frustration was summed up by a British physician, Sir Thomas Lewis: "Reflection tells me that I am so far from being able to satisfactorily define pain that the attempt would serve no useful purpose. Pain, like similar subjective things, is known to us by experience and described by illustration."

The inability of doctor and philosopher alike to describe pain satisfactorily was matched, historically, by their inability until very recent times to do much about relieving it.

The desperation of patients seeking relief may be inferred from the lengths to which they went to achieve it in medieval times. In England, powdered moss, grown on a human skull, was taken like snuff to serve as a pain killer. A variety of endless chants were used, and villagers would chew almost anything not immediately poisonous if anyone could be found who would claim it had pain-killing properties. Yet chants had only the power of suggestion to support them, while only those herbal cures based on drug-bearing plants (a slim minority) achieved much effect.

But as unpleasant as pain is, we would not be better off if it could somehow be eliminated. Pain serves as an indicator of disease and injury. Without it, children would not learn so quickly to avoid fire, adults would be unable to tell when their teeth were decayed, and everyone would have a far more difficult time detecting the onset of illness or injury.

Persons who cannot feel pain, usually as the result of spinal or brain injuries, face special problems. A prominent example is Alabama Gov. George Wallace, numb from the waist down because of spinal damage after an assassination attempt. During the 1976 presidential campaign, his leg was accidentally broken by aides removing him from an aircraft. His risk of serious infection was great, because the break went undiscovered for days after it happened. Eventually, the break was indicated by swelling. Pain, were it possible, would have resulted in immediate discovery and reduced hazard.

Types of Pain

Many theories of pain abound, dividing the sensation into categories of pricking pain, aching, clear and quick pain, but most researchers accept a general division into aching and pricking pain. Pricking pain is felt in the skin, muscles, and bones—sharp and insistent—often throbbing with the heartbeat. Aching pain is sensed in the internal organs, such as stomach, throat, or appendix, and does not generally throb. Unlike pricking pain, aching pain is not usually limited to the specific area of its source; often, one's brain "reports" the pain as coming from the skin area above the organ involved.

Different types of pain are survival mechanisms that evolved from the simplest organisms. In order to survive without intelligence, a creature must respond to external pain in one fashion, internal pain in another. External pain may often be avoided by flight; but running away aggravates pain from within, since it usually results from diseased or damaged tissue, muscle, joints, or bones.

A bee sting or an enemy's arrow would be *external* pain

51

sources, resulting in pricking pain. Either would elicit the "flight-fight" response. The appropriate response to a pricking pain is either escape or fight. The body prepares by releasing extra adrenalin, increasing a person's energy, strength, and sensitivity to pain.

Pricking pain is also location-specific—the pain of a cracked funnybone or sore shoulder muscle. The ability to locate this kind of pain is important, so the specific injured area can be favored.

Diseased or damaged tissue, *interal* pain sources, more often result in aching pain, which causes a person to slow down. Running from an inflamed appendix is not helpful. Aching pain is deep and persistent and results in lethargy, depression, and reduced movement, which provides the body a chance to mend the damage at its source. The source is not important to the reaction, so the inability of aching pain to pinpoint location is insignificant.

Physical Versus Psychological

Pain has both a physical and a psychological effect on its victim. Aspirin primarily affects the physical response, but to understand the effect, pain perception must also be understood.

Pain is perceived physically at nerve endings and registered in the brain. The first link is physical, one of chemicals and cells, and is well understood; the second is psychological and, as with most matters of perception, is poorly understood.

Pain is felt when nerve endings are stimulated by chemicals released from nearby cells. These cells can be triggered to release the pain-causing chemical bradykinin by physical stimuli, such as penetration of a bee's stinger, or chemical stimuli, such as the by-products of a disease process. If there is enough bradykinin near the end of a nerve, it will send out a pain message. Slightly smaller amounts will produce a tickling sensation.

Coming in from the extremities, the nerves are bundled together into the spinal cord. According to scientists who study pain (dolorologists), the body may choose to cut off the pain impulse at the spinal cord. This "pain gate" mechanism can either be operated by the nerves themselves (shutting out minor pain until it becomes major) or by the mind (for reasons noted later). But if the pain gets through the gate, it is routed to the thalamus, where the physical act of pain perception is completed.

The thalamus sorts out pain impulses, determines their origins and severity, and sends the information to the cortex.

Pain has its psychological effect in the cortex, the thinking, feeling part of the brain. Once the cortex has been offered a pain perception, it may choose a variety of reactions. Fatigue, fear, anxiety, and the anticipation of more pain are known to intensify pain reactions; joy and a sense of relief reduce them. Reactions can also vary with age, sex, cultural background, and upbringing and are known to vary from day to day within the same person.

Since pain is registered in the thinking part of the brain, it can just as readily be the result of imagination as of a physical stimulus. On occasion, pain is felt in the absence of any disease or injury and examination reveals no chemical stimulus of nerve endings. In such cases, dolorologists suspect projection of emotions, perhaps anxiety or guilt, in the form of pain, onto particular parts of the body, in a purely psychological process.

Aspirin Fights Pain

Chemically, aspirin blocks the physical perception of pain through chemical action; psychologically, it can sometimes erase the registration of pain in the cortex, through the power of suggestion.

Different types of pain result from different types of chemical stimulation. When pain is the result of disease or internal injury, there is a constant flow of pain-causing bradykinin. Pain caused by an external injury usually leads to a momentary burst of chemical release.

Pricking pain continues after the first burst because tiny amounts of bradykinin are aided by "magnifier" hormones (described later in this chapter) released as part of the bodily reaction to injury. Aspirin blocks magnifier release at the nerve endings and in the thalamus, where magnifiers assist in pain interpretation, cutting pain off at both ends of its physical path. Aching pain is generally caused by a continuous chemical release, so magnifiers play a smaller role and aspirin is less effective in reducing it.

Imaginary pain is relieved by aspirin through the power of suggestion, despite the lack of any known physical effect in such cases. Suffering is also psychological and is the end result of pain; this makes assessment of the next pain-blocking effect of aspirin very difficult, since highly variable non-physical conditions play a major role in the patient's response to pain.

This variability and the power of suggestion make pain relievers difficult to test. As many as 35 percent of the participants in some studies report significant pain reduction from a placebo, a harmless sugar pill disguised as a drug.

If a person believes aspirin works, it usually has some effect on almost any kind of pain, although the same could be said of any pill the patient believed in. Aspirin has proven most effective for the types of pain it provably interferes with, including headaches, muscle pains, tooth extractions, and impacted wisdom teeth. Any pain-causing injury that also involves inflammation is doubly susceptible to treatment with aspirin, since the drug reduces inflammation as well as pain.

Fever and Inflammation

Inflammation is a sign of your body's defensive systems at work. Its symptoms are pain, redness, swelling, and hot skin. Inflammation can be caused by diseases or injury, may be a factor in some headaches and usually accompanies muscular pain. Inflammation is more fully discussed in Chapter 5, since it is a major symptom of arthritis.

Chronic inflammation is an overreaction of the body's immune system, often aggravated by the same magnifier hormone that makes nerve endings more sensitive to bradykinin. By blocking production of this magnifier, aspirin reduces inflammation.

Fever is also a sign of the body's defenses at work; white blood cells, destroyed while repelling microbes, release pyrogens, or fever-causing chemicals. These pyrogens are carried in the blood to a brain section called the hypothalamus—the body's thermostat—where they increase body temperature to aid the white cells, which fight infection more effectively in a warmer body.

Fever not only helps mobilize bodily defenses, it also causes discomfort in adults and convulsions in children, so doctors sometimes prescribe aspirin to reduce the risk of side effects.

Aspirin chemically resets the hypothalamus by blocking creation of the "magnifier" hormone triggered by incoming pyrogens. If there are no pyrogens, there are no magnifiers, so the hypothalamus temperature setting is unaffected, which explains why aspirin reduces fevers, but not normal temperatures.

When aspirin lowers fever, however, it does not rid the body of the excess heat used to battle disease. The hypothalamus controls heat production and heat loss; pyrogens only turn up heat production, leaving losses constant. Aspirin resets the loss side, increasing heat radiation through sweating and extra blood flow in the skin.

Because there is some decrease in heat available to help the immune system when aspirin lowers fever, it is seldom prescribed for fevers below 101 in adults. Children are prone to convulsions and brain damage during most fevers, so aspirin is prescribed more often for their fevers.

Untreated Causes

The advancing stages of many diseases often go unnoticed if their symptoms are masked by aspirin. Pain, fever, and inflammation, sometimes seemingly minor, may be the only signal of an internal problem. The AMA *Drug Evaluations* suggests doctors prescribing aspirin for fever "find and cure the cause," since symptom reduction removes the patient's sense of urgency about finding the cause. Masking of pain and inflammation is also a problem; the onslaught of arthritis is marked by inflammation and, as noted, pain is the precursor of many conditions.

Sometimes the line between symptom reduction for minor ailments and symptom masking for life-threatening disease is a hard one to draw. Take, for example, the relief of headache pain, aspirin's second most common use after relief of arthritis symptoms. About 3.5 million persons, 1.5 percent of the population, suffer from headaches during a given week; the vast majority are minor, a handful are life-threatening.

A pioneer in headache study, the late Harold G. Wolff, described two kinds of headaches, intercranial and extracranial. Migraine, tension, and sinus headaches are medically less serious extracranial headaches. Migraines involve changes in blood vessels, and usually throb in tempo with the heartbeat. Tension headaches are centered in the neck and scalp muscles, but are often perceived in the forehead and base of the neck. Sinus headaches accompany allergies or infections of the nose and sinuses and produce pain in the forehead and near the eyes.

Intercranial headaches are more serious, often resulting from infections or tumors and, if untreated, can cause serious injury or death. As a rule, they do not throb, but hurt continuously, with more intensity in the morning, and may be associated with nausea.

Evolving Theory

Tracking down the mechanism of aspirin's operation was a complicated task, which took nearly three-quarters of a century to complete. Certainly Dr. Felix Hoffman, the man who discovered the effects of aspirin, had no inkling how it worked; all he knew for certain was it relieved his father's agonizing pain and seemed to have few side effects.

It was easier to trace the operation of other drugs, which had more specific effects; if they affected the kidney, for example, their concentration there could be detected, their effect minutely examined. But aspirin's effects are spread throughout the body; in the brain, in joint and muscle tissues, in the nervous system. Reduction of pain, fever, and inflammation are seemingly unrelated processes, so researchers wondered how one drug could achieve these effects.

Studies on humans indicated pain effects at the nerve end and thalamus, fever reduction at the hypothalamus and inflammation discouraged, whatever its location. Although aspirin's physical ends were known in the 1940's, its means remained a mystery.

By 1963, Dr. Harry Collier, of the British branch of Miles Laboratories, had developed a theory of aspirin operation that pinpointed the immune system as the source of the symptoms it relieved. In the *Scientific American* of October, 1963, he postulated an "anti-defensive" role for aspirin, suggesting it checked an over-exuberance on the part of the immune system during its defense against disease.

"It would appear that the human body has an unwieldy defense establishment that aspirin fortunately can help control," Collier wrote.

Prostaglandins: They're Everywhere

Assuming aspirin achieves its effects through control of a single family of chemicals, these chemicals would have to be found everywhere in the body. Chemicals in the immune system meet that requirement, but aspirin seemed to have scant effect on chemicals that circulate through the bloodstream. The discovery of aspirin's method of operation was not possible until the discovery of chemicals formed, used and broken down quickly near the cells that created them.

The pain and inflammation magnifying chemicals, also present in the hypothalamus during fever, are just such a group; they are called prostaglandins (PG's). These hormones are regulators, starting and stopping various body functions. PG's play a regulatory role in many places, including the reproductive system, the stomach, the intestines, the bloodstream, the heart, the nervous system, the lungs, and the kidney.

In some cases, PG's can both start and stop a function; a small amount serves as a trigger, increasing amounts act as a magnifier until the function peaks, then gross amounts stop the function.

Although study of PG's began with their discovery in 1930, the research did not reach fruition until the late 1960's. The link between aspirin and prostaglandins was not as long in coming, but it took two years, from 1969 until 1971, to forge it.

The aspirin-PG relationship is just one small part of the most promising, wide-open field of medical research today, prostaglandin research. The more than twenty hormones in this chemical family may be the most minutely studied group of substances medical science has ever known; they are ubiquitous and powerful even in doses of one ten-billionth of an ounce. Cells create PG's in such small amounts for specific tasks: once the task is performed, the PG breaks down and disappears, sometimes in as little as thirty seconds.

One method used to study PG effects is to give aspirin when PG's are suspected of causing a symptom. If the symptom is alleviated, PG's become a prime suspect. Aspirin halts PG production as effectively as almost any other drug, for periods ranging from minutes in some cells to days in others.

PG History

The subtlety of PG's—short life, minute amounts—contributed to the great length of time it took to understand and appreciate them. With crude instruments, medical science began to unlock the secrets of grosser internal human chemical reactions at the end of the nineteenth century. Knowledge about body chemistry grew, as did the sophistication of the tools used to seek further information. It seems unlikely we will ever know how all parts of the body function, but there were certainly fewer unknowns by 1930 then there had been at the turn of the century.

Discovery of a new chemical group, which would, as a by-product, eventually explain the operation of aspirin, was not the goal of gynecologist Dr. Rapheal Kurzok, or pharmacologist Charles C. Lieb, in 1930. They were performing artificial insemination in a New York City clinic when they found women were uncomfortable during insemination because of occasional uterine wall contractions.

Experimenting on samples of uterine muscle tissue, the pair isolated a substance in human sperm that seemed to cause the contractions. Another researcher, Ulf S. von Euler, concluded the substance was produced by the prostate gland, so it was called prostaglandin. This misnamed hormone, actually a whole group of hormones, was given credit primarily for the sole side effect that led to its discovery and was to be roundly ignored by most researchers for thirty years.

The early discovery of PG's was made possible by their high concentration in semen, the highest concentration anywhere in the body. The later discovery of their presence elsewhere was impossible until development of instruments refined enough to detect PG's in minute quantities.

Early research was also stymied by the small amounts of naturally occuring PG's. Between their discovery in 1930 and the exploding volume of research in the mid-1960's, an average of only one scientific paper a year was written about prostaglandins. Presently, the increased level of scientific interest and experimentation is shown by the publication of about three PG papers every day!

The difference in interest resulted from a turnaround in the PG supply situation, from scarcity to abundance. During the 1940's and 1950's, tons of sheep semen had to be gathered to produce a usable quantity of PG's. Then, working in Sweden's Karolinska Institute in 1965, Dr. Sune Bergstrom developed a method of biosynthesis, at the same time it was discovered in the United States by The Upjohn Co. and in Holland by Unilever. The discovery was as important as Kolbe's synthesis, 100 years earlier, of salicylic acid (SA). Researchers explored SA as fast as it could be synthesized, eventually discovering aspirin; in the same way, biosynthesis of PG's freed researchers from dependence on expensive natural PG's. In fact, to encourage PG research, Upjohn provides free PG samples to researchers. This new availability led to the discovery of PG's relationship to aspirin, among other drugs.

Discovery of the Connection

Dr. John Vane discovered the connection between aspirin and prostaglandins following the research begun by one of his graduate students in 1969, when he was in the pharmacology department of the Royal College of Surgeons in London. Vane is now a research scientist at the British laboratories of Burroughs-Wellcome, a pharmaceutical manufacturer. During a November, 1976, visit to the United States, he described the discovery process to the author.

In 1969, working jointly with graduate student Priscilla Piper, Vane discovered a substance that made rabbit blood vessels contract. Their original discovery echoed that of Kurzok and Lieb in 1930; they presumed the substance had only a single effect. But continuing work soon convinced them they had found a prostaglandin.

Vane says the research then took an unplanned turn. Piper had worked at a pharmaceutical firm before joining him; she had developed an interest in aspirin and was looking for an aspirin-PG link. Vane describes what happened next:

> I remember on that occasion, in 1971, I had the idea over the weekend. I called Priscilla and all my colleagues and said, "I think I know how aspirin works. Do You?" They all said no. I said, "I am going off to do an experiment." By lunch time, I had done the experiment and it worked.

Vane had proven, to his own satisfaction, that aspirin worked by stopping bodily production of prostaglandins. Aspirin's ability to reduce fever, pain, and inflammation stems from its PG effect, according to Vane and others. There are "one or two pockets of resistance" to the PG explanation of aspirin's effects, Vane said, but he added, "They aren't very active."

How Aspirin Works

Aspirin works by preventing the body's production of PG's, normally produced by enzymes triggered by an activator. A PG enzyme, when triggered, takes arachadonic acid from cell walls and combines it with oxygen and other substances to make a PG. Chemically, aspirin (an acid) takes the place of arachadonic acid on the enzyme, preventing PG synthesis.

How are pain, fever, and inflammation reduced by reduction of PG synthesis? In the preceeding description of these symptoms, "magnifier" hormones played significant roles: these hormones are prostaglandins, and in their absence all three symptoms are reduced in intensity or eliminated.

Aspirin, in addition to quelling these symptoms, increases the amount of time blood takes to clot, again by reducing the rate at which PG's are produced. Prostaglandins contribute to the clotting process by allowing platelets in the blood to stick more easily to each other and to blood vessel walls. These platelets form the basis of clots in arteries; in the presence of PG's, it takes only a small stimulus to form a platelet plug. When PG formation is blocked by aspirin, plugs still form, but nowhere near as readily. Clots formed by weak stimuli are believed to play a role in heart attacks and strokes. If aspirin can reduce the incidence of these unwanted clots, it may reduce the incidence of these two diseases, a promising possibility that is discussed in Chapter 7.

New Aspirin Uses

With the newly accepted explanation of how aspirin works, medical researchers can now predict the effects of aspirin in any process or disease in which PG's play a role.

For example, some cancer patients, especially those with cancer of the lung, breast, or kidney, have higher than normal amounts of calcium in their blood. This condition, known as hypercalcemia, may result from increased prostaglandin production that has been triggered by cancer cells. Hypercalcemia causes vomiting, loss of appetite, delusions, and lethargy.

At Vanderbilt University Medical School in Nashville, researchers gave patients with cancer-induced hypercalcemia between four and fifteen aspirin tablets a day as treatment. The patients' blood calcium level dropped, supporting the theory that cancer caused hypercalcemia by raising PG levels in the body. When aspirin treatment was halted, calcium levels rose again.

Cancer tumors apparently raise the PG level in order to insure their own survival. The body's immune system normally attacks cancer cells, but does so less efficiently at high PG levels. Prostaglandin supression of the immune system is often fought with indomethicin, a drug that works slightly better than aspirin in preventing formation of PG's, but which has more side effects. If eventually proved out, PG-blocking drugs would probably not be a complete cancer treatment, but may be useful in connection with other cancer therapies.

The role of PG's in reproduction is indicated by their natural abundance in semen, where they are observed in unusually large concentrations. It is now believed that reduced PG levels may lead to male infertility, an assumption that is the basis of research on development of a male birth-control pill.

Dr. William S. Fields of the University of Texas at Houston told the author of an observation he has made, but never published. Poor women in the Southwest and in Puerto Rico use aspirin as a contraceptive, although the method has never, to his knowledge, been tested or proven. But these women believe insertion of an aspirin tablet prior to intercourse will prevent conception.

PG research casts doubt on this particular folklore. PG's are believed to trigger menstruation, and inter-uterine birth-control devices (IUD's) are thought to take advantage of this by stimulating PG production and menstruation, even when an egg has been fertilized. Some doctors now believe that the occasional failure of an IUD may be explained by unwitting consumption of aspirin, or other PG-blocking drugs.

On the other hand, PG's in excessive amounts have been shown to play a role in menstrual disorders. Taking aspirin, or aspirin compounds, to relieve menstrual pain (under such brand names as Midol) may not only relieve pain, it may relieve the cause of the pain, which is excessive PG production.

In other reproduction-PG research, at the Postgraduate Medical School in Budapest, Hungary, doctors have used sodium salicylate, an aspirin-like drug, to prevent preterm abortion and delivery caused by premature uterine activity. A normal pregnancy requires a balance between female hormones and PG hormones. If the hormone level drops, the PG level must also be cut. In fifty women tested, uterine activity halted within eight hours after a ten-tablet dose of the aspirin-like drug reduced PG levels. Other treatments were then used to restore the PG-female-hormone balance.

The experiments mentioned are just a sampling of the research going on in the area of prostaglandins, much of which also involves aspirin, the safest of the drugs that effectively halt PG production. Much work on PG's is ongoing and much remains to be done: they are likely to provide medical science with its greatest challenge and most challenging opportunity in the years to come.

5

Aspirin and Arthritis

Arthritis may well be the oldest chronic affliction on earth. Signs of the disease have been found in dinosaur remains; it is believed to have afflicted Henry VI, Charlemagne, Alexander the Great, and Goethe.

The word "arthritis" itself literally means inflammation of a joint. "Arthritis" is loosely used to refer to more than 100 diseases that involve some degree of inflammation. In general, it appears that the greater role inflammation plays in an arthritic disease, the greater benefit obtained by taking aspirin. Treatment of the two most common forms of arthritis, osteoarthritis and rheumatoid arthritis, nearly always involves aspirin.

If fact, the need for effective treatment of rheumatoid arthritis led directly to Dr. Felix Hoffman's discovery of the effects of aspirin, when his father became unable to tolerate then-available pain killers.

To reduce the pain and inflammation that are symptoms of arthritis, doctors usually prescribe as much aspirin as an arthritic can tolerate, often 20 tablets a day, or 7,000 tablets a year. More than 20 million Americans are under medical treatment for arthritis, including 12 million with osteoarthritis and 5 million with rheumatoid arthritis; all told, arthritics take half the aspirin consumed in the United States.

There are 600,000 new cases of arthritis reported each year and its total cost to the community at large is estimated at $13 billion. More than 3.5 million persons in the United States have been crippled, totally or in part, by forms of arthritis.

Although there are 20 million persons being treated for arthritis, the government estimates another 30 million persons have less troublesome cases. Many of these persons have arthritis that could be detected by special tests, but which presently manifests only minor symptoms.

Governmental and private agencies spend less than $30 million each year on arthritis research and prevention, a miniscule figure compared to the disease's estimated costs: included in the $13 billion total is $4.8 billion in lost wages, $1.5 billion in hospital costs, $1.4 billion in lost homemaker services, $1 billion in insurance losses and at least another $1.5 billion on medication.

Who Has Arthritis?

During the 1960s, the U.S. Department of Health, Education, and Welfare conducted a study of the incidence of arthritis. HEW found 154 persons out of 1,000 above the age of forty-five believed they had arthritis; below age forty-five, the figure was 15 out of 1,000.

The agency found 10 persons out of 1,000 had clear cases of rheumatoid arthritis, while a surprising 22 out of 1,000 showed "probable" signs of the disease. Arthritis is more common among the elderly and, inexplicably, is three times as common among women as among men.

Although some elderly persons have rheumatoid arthritis, most suffer from osteoarthritis, or degenerative joint disease. It is believed that this breakdown of joint tissue is a natural part of the aging process and cannot be prevented: it afflicts men and women in equal numbers. Although 97 percent of all persons over the age of sixty have osteoarthritis, which is visible on X-rays, not all of them suffer from its symptoms of joint pain and immobility.

What Is Arthritis?

Arthritis is a chronic process that is perfectly normal in its short-term appearances: inflammation.

Inflammation is triggered when the body is injured, or invaded by foreign material, such as a virus, bacteria, or toxic inanimate material. Chronic inflammation has the same origins, but is uncontrolled, continuing long after the original stimulus has departed.

Inflammation indicates your body is protecting itself from disease or damage by activating its immune system. This system is comprised of cells and chemicals in the blood that fight "alien" materials, animate or inanimate matter the immune system detects as not being part of the body.

Scientists know which stimuli cause normal inflammation; injury, disease or foreign matter. They are uncertain why these stimuli sometimes trigger chronic inflammation.

One prominent theory suggests chronic inflammation is begun by a bacteria so powerful it triggers an overreaction by the immune system. Another theory states that body cells themselves are changed by a viral or chemical reaction, in a fashion that makes them appear foreign to the immune system. This "autoimmune" response can, if unchecked, result in people literally developing an immunity to parts of their own body, such as joints. The result can be uncontrolled inflammation, that is, arthritis.

When a body cell is attacked by disease or injury, it releases chemicals that attract white blood cells. These white cells then attempt to destroy the invading material. If the source of chronic inflammation is a virus, as some scientists believe, white cells destroy the virus before it can be examined.

As an area of the body becomes filled with the chemical by-products of white cells, some of them release lysosomal enzymes.

These are very potent and are normally used inside white cells to destroy waste material and debris. When these enzymes are released, they destroy body cells, making the nearby area warm, red, and painful; in short, inflammed.

If arthritis is not stopped, it can manifest itself throughout the body, attacking joints and internal organs far from its original site. This occurs via intervention of chemicals known as antibodies, formed in the blood. Antibodies attach themselves to foreign matter and attract white cells to destroy it: they travel through the blood, looking for foreign matter similar to that they were created to attack. If antibodies are created that attack joint tissue—because the joint tissue has been altered to appear foreign—they will attach to it anywhere in the body. Antibodies in turn attract white cells, which destroy the joint tissue. Since blood vessels, lungs, and the kidney are made of the same kind of tissue as joints, they can also become inflammed by arthritis.

Major types of arthritis that primarily create inflammation include rheumatoid arthritis, aklyosing spondylitis, rheumatic fever, and gout. Dozens of more obscure forms also involve the process described.

Osteoarthritis

The most common form of arthritis, osteoarthritis, however, involves inflammation only peripherally, as an effect, rather than a cause.

Osteoarthritis is primarily a disease of the elderly; most persons over the age of sixty show signs of osteoarthritis' deterioration in X-rays of their joints, but many do not feel its symptoms. Osteoarthritis is also known as degenerative joint disease and is primarily the result of physical stress on the joints. It is usually found in the knee or hip and sometimes involves inflammation.

Other factors besides age seem to influence the onset and course of the disease, which can manifest itself as early as age forty. Some persons have hereditary tendencies to osteoarthritis, others are struck at a younger age than normal because they use a single joint to excess; ballet dancers, for example, get it in their ankles, athletes in various joints. Injuries can also lead to a sudden manifestation of osteoarthritis.

In short, osteoarthritis is primarily a disease of wear and tear, striking mainly the elderly, with a fairly well understood set of causes. Rheumatoid arthritis, as well as most other forms of the disease, can strike at any age and is more varied in origin.

Arthritis Treatment

All major forms of arthritis respond to treatment with aspirin, which is the backbone of most programs of arthritis therapy. The object of drug therapy in treatment of arthritis is to reduce pain and inflammation and prevent further joint damage. Many more expensive drugs, with higher risk of side effects, are used for these purposes, but none has proven more effective and safer than aspirin. There, is, however, no "cure" for arthritis, and not likely to be one, until its sources are better understood.

For the time being, researchers are focusing both on prevention and control. Their success in control has been significant; medically supervised aspirin-taking, while it does nothing for damage already caused, prevents further joint destruction by reducing inflammation. It also makes damage that occurred prior to treatment more tolerable by reducing its pain.

Aspirin controls inflammation because it controls bodily production of prostaglandins (PG's), which play a role in *starting* and *stopping* normal inflammation.

Outbreaks of inflammation that halt themselves are the rule, rather than the exception. Inflammation is usually a four-stage process, as described before.

First, the cells under attack give off chemicals that attract the immune system.

Second, if the disease or injury is major, the number of white cells in the area increases until lysosomal enzymes are released.

Third, those enzymes destroy body cells, releasing chemicals from the cell walls. One chemical is the base for PG creation. PG's cause pain, redness, and swelling and attract more white cells. In small amounts, PG's promote inflammation.

Fourth, large amounts of PG's are eventually produced; such amounts discourage further inflammation by decreasing the release of chemicals that attract white cells. PG's in large amounts also discourage white cells already in the area from releasing more lysosomal enzymes. When the fourth, self-regulating stage does not occur, arthritis is often the result.

Body cells, unassisted by PG's, can create only small amounts of inflammation. By supressing PG production, aspirin can reduce inflammation in the third stage of the process.

PG control can also directly reduce the crippling effects of rheumatoid arthritis. Joints in the fingers, wrists, hands, feet, and toes are commonly affected, becoming swollen, tender, and painful. The symptoms indicate the cartilage found at the junctions of bones is being destroyed. Without drugs, therapy, or both, this destruction can result in scar tissue, which eventually turns to bone, fusing the joint together and making it immobile.

Prostaglandins assist this progression from destruction to scar tissue to bone; their absence can slow it. Thus, taking aspirin can substantially reduce the loss of joint mobility, which often accompanies many forms of arthritis.

Because PG production must be constantly reduced, aspirin prescriptions for arthritis differ from those for pain. For pain, the dose is usually two tablets. For arthritis, the dose is gradually increased until the patient shows early signs of aspirin poisoning, including ringing ears. The dose is then reduced to the maximum tolerable level below that; up to twenty aspirin tablets a day. The AMA's *Drug Evaluations* estimates 90 percent of all minor cases of arthritis can be treated in this fashion.

Acetaminophen (Tylenol, Datril) is rarely prescribed for arthritis. Although it relieves pain, it has no effect on inflammation. In those rare cases in which a person cannot tolerate aspirin, other, riskier, non-aspirin drugs are used.

Osteoarthritis Treatment

At the present time, aspirin is used in osteoarthritis treatment to reduce pain and inflammation, while efforts are made to reduce the stress on affected joints, through weight loss or rest. But a wider role for aspirin has been predicted.

A landmark paper describing this prospect was written in 1972, by Dr. O. Donald Chrisman of Yale, for the journal *Clinical Orthopaedics and Related Research*. He wrote that osteoarthritis may not be solely the result of joint wear, but might be caused in part by "softening" of joint cartilage.

When deterioration occurs faster than tissue renewal, cartilage softens, Chrisman found. He proposed slowing degeneration, so regeneration could keep up or get ahead.

Aspirin gives the body the edge it needs to overcome softened cartilage; in rabbits, it slowed softening by 20 percent. He tested the theory on humans with dislocated knee caps, giving 36 patients 10 tablets daily for up to 8 weeks. Only 14 took aspirin; the rest received placebos. Patients were not randomly distributed into the two groups and the doctors knew, although the patients didn't, who got aspirin and who didn't.

Among the non-aspirin patients, of 23 knees examined, 21 showed some sign of softening. Among aspirin patients, only 3 of 16 knees examined showed softening. The odds of this result occuring by chance are 1 in 10,000.

Aspirin will not "turn back the clock" and repair damage already done; it must be started within a few days after dislocation in order to be effective, Chrisman wrote.

As with rheumatoid arthritis and other related forms, no preventative treatment is yet known for osteoarthritis. Unlike the other forms, aspirin alone is not presently believed to arrest osteoarthritis' progress; its spread is halted only through stress reduction at joints.

Other Major Forms

The numbers of persons affected by the three other major members of the arthritis family are difficult to estimate. Rheumatic fever afflicts thousands each year, usually children between the ages of five and fifteen. It often causes temporary cases of severe arthritis and sometimes permanent heart damage. Gout, which has arthritis as a symptom, afflicts men several times more often than women, for unknown reasons; about 2 persons out of 1,000 can expect to have gout during their lifetime. Anklyosing spondylitis strikes about 1 person out of 2,000, is often undiagnosed and typically afflicts men between the ages of fifteen and forty.

All three diseases are painful and are sometimes self-treated with aspirin. Although aspirin has some utility in treatment of these diseases, its use to control them without medical supervision is risky and can be counterproductive.

About three million persons have undiagnosed cases of ankylosing spondylitis, according to the Arthritis Foundation. The disease is often hereditary and rarely manifests itself after age thirty. Lower back pain, eye inflammation or hip and shoulder pain are symptoms; curvature of the spine can result if treatment is delayed. Physical therapy and prescriptions of aspirin are the standard treatment.

Gout, or gouty arthritis as it is sometimes known, is a painful disease caused by excess levels of uric acid—a body waste product —in the blood. Gout was once thought to be caused by rich food, but researchers now believe a person must be predisposed to gout in order to have an attack. Attacks may occur with or without obvious stimulus, but are sometimes brought on by eating crab, liver, kidneys, or sweetbreads. Joint pain, usually in the large joint of the big toe, results from uric acid crystals forming in the joints. The crystals trigger an immune reaction and inflammation.

For several decades after its discovery, large doses of aspirin were used to reduce uric acid levels but other more specific drugs have supplanted aspirin. Caution should be used when taking it in small doses to relieve the pain of gout; in small doses, aspirin increases uric acid levels, interfering with other drugs used to treat the disease.

Rheumatic fever is classed with arthritis because it involves inflammation. The inflammation stimulus is streptococcus bacteria, and the symptoms are fever and arthritis. Rheumatic fever is treated with antibiotics to end the infection and aspirin to control the fever and arthritis, and to reduce the extra burden these symptoms place on the heart. Permanent heart damage can be the end result of rheumatic fever, and the disease is sometimes fatal. The AMA "Primer on the Rheumatic Diseases" declares aspirin sometimes "tilt[s] the balance in favor of survival of a more critically ill patient."

Symptoms and Diagnosis

Arthritis is a difficult disease for both patients and doctors to deal with, because in its early stages, before major damage has been done, its symptoms are minor and easily controlled by aspirin, or ignored entirely.

Aches and pains can mean many things, but a doctor should be consulted if the following symptoms persist:

1. pain and stiffness when waking;
2. pain or tenderness in one or more joints;
3. swelling in one or more joints;
4. recurrence of symptoms, especially in one or more joints;
5. noticeable pain and stiffness in the lower back, knees, or other joints;
6. tingling sensation in the fingertips, hands, and feet;
7. unexplained weight loss, fever, weakness or fatigue.

Although early diagnosis of the disease is difficult, it is also important. The earlier that arthritis is detected, the earlier it can be controlled; proper control will often provide substantial reduction in joint damage.

A doctor obviously cannot diagnose arthritis if the patient remains unexamined. Some arthritics waited as long as four years from the first appearance of symptoms before seeking professional help. On the other hand, it is inadvisable to run to the doctor every time one awakens with stiff joints. Specialists suggest a visit to the doctor if symptoms persist for six weeks or more.

The Nature of Arthritis

Arthritis differs from the diseases most people are used to dealing with; those that come, incapacitate for a week or two and then are gone. Colds and flu, the most common diseases, are of this type. Arthritis and related diseases are different; once manifested, they frequently continue for a lifetime. They are chronic, and the medical science of 1977 cannot cure them; all it can do is control them and reduce the damage they do.

If you have a chronic disease like arthritis, you must expect to change the way you live in order to deal with it, possibly for decades. Whether the doctor finds you need medication, exercise, or both (in some cases, even surgery), often the most you can hope for is that your arthritis will not get worse.

Sometimes arthritis will seem better, even if you do not take the aspirin or other drug your doctor prescribes; or its symptoms will lessen if you take large, unprescribed doses of aspirin. This reduction of symptoms is one of the frustrating aspects of arthritis treatment, because these short periods of time in which symptoms seem to disappear do not mean the disease is cured. These remissions, as they are called, can occur whether the disease is being treated or not.

Arthritis is known for frequent remissions, often lasting weeks or even years. About 10 percent of the time the symptoms never recur, although the damage done to joints is permanent and remains. In 90 percent of all cases, the symptoms do return, often worse than before. Without a doctor's approval, patients should not discontinue treatment simply because the symptoms of arthritis have disappeared.

Arthritis Treatment

Arthritis Foundation figures show fraudulent or "quack" products are almost as widely used as reliable non-prescription drugs for treatment of arthritis. When a person experiences reduced symptoms after using a "quack" drug, he or she will usually attribute improvement to the drug, not to a spontaneous remission. Quackery is expensive; in addition to relieving victims of $485 million a year, it often delays treatment, thus aggravating problems and pain, in the long run.

Self-diagnosis and treatment are obviously a poor idea. You cannot tell what kind of arthritis you have, or how much aspirin (or other drugs) to take for it without laboratory tests and a thorough examination by a qualified physician.

There are still people who believe diet and climate are the keys to controlling or even curing arthritis, but scientific evidence is overwhelmingly against these factors. There is no evidence the disease itself becomes less destructive in a warm climate, although the sufferer may often feel better there. There is also no scientific evidence any food or vitamin deficiency has anything to do with causing arthritis or can help reduce its course or its pain.

There are drugs that can control arthritis, however.

Some of them are new and expensive (as much as ten cents per dose, compared to one cent or less for aspirin); more new ones are being discovered constantly. Despite the enormous amount of money poured into research and testing of new and more powerful arthritis treatments, both Consumers Union and the AMA's "Primer" agree aspirin is the first drug a doctor should prescribe for the two major forms of arthritis, osteoarthritis and rheumatoid arthritis, which account for 85 percent of all arthritis victims.

Self-Medication and Advertising

The Arthritis Foundation is concerned about aspirin advertising, because it believes the general tone plays down the seriousness of arthritis. The organization concedes, of course, that aspirin is a tremendously effective drug for the treatment of arthritis, but only under medical supervision. The foundation objects to the depiction of common rheumatoid arthritis or osteoarthritis as a disease of minor aches, although manufacturers contend their advertisements are merely advising that aspirin self-medication be limited to mild pain. The foundation stated, "The truth is, arthritis can be a serious disease. The pain can be excruciating and the results can be severe crippling unless the victim starts full and proper medical treatment in the early stages."

In addition, the Arthritis Foundation told a Food and Drug Administration panel, "Self-medication may lead to delay in seeking medical attention until after preventable joint damage has taken place. Arthritis sufferers would be best served if the word 'arthritis' were banned from aspirin product labeling and advertising, leaving the medication decision to physicians."

Doctors who treat arthritis say their patients often refuse to believe that aspirin is going to be effective in controlling the disease. Many patients question how anything so commonly used could be good for such a painful and long-term illness. But aspirin's prevalence stems in part from its effectiveness. The AMA *Drug Evaluations* suggests aspirin be prescribed even when more powerful and expensive anti-arthritic drugs are prescribed, in order to reduce the doses of the more powerful drugs and minimize side effects.

Long-Term Treatment

When medical attention is sought in connection with arthritis, aspirin is often the prescription. Once the doctor is convinced aspirin will work, there is still the problem of continuing the drug program and dampening fears of an accidental overdose.

Large-dose aspirin therapy is usually long-term, but doctors administering it run into problems with their patients, who will not take it when their pain is gone. Few patients seem to realize the drug is being used not only to fight pain, but to reduce inflammation, and must be maintained at all times in the bloodstream. Otherwise, its anti-inflammatory effect is drastically weakened.

Doctors administering aspirin for arthritis have noted a decreased frequency of heart attacks and strokes among those taking large doses for long periods of time, relative to the general, non-aspirin-taking public. This effect was not immediately attributed to aspirin because doctors could not conceive how the drug could have such an effect.

Aspirin use by arthritics and observation by doctors, together with prostaglandin research, gave rise to a plausible theory explaining aspirin's ability to reduce the risk of heart attack and stroke. The testing of that theory is well underway, if not yet completed, as we will describe in Chapter 7.

6

Aspirin Side Effects

All drugs have side effects and aspirin is no exception. When it is taken to produce one effect and produces an undesired one, aspirin causes side effects. Such side effects are typically related to the amount of aspirin taken and the frequency of doses. Side effects are more likely and more severe if the dose is more than three tablets or is taken more frequently than once every four hours.

The side effects of aspirin are rare, relative to those of most other effective drugs. This is not to say there is no risk involved in taking aspirin; at normal doses, the most common side effects are upset stomach and undetectable stomach bleeding. Much rarer are allergic reaction and temporary deafness.

In overdose, aspirin is dangerous, as are all over-the-counter drugs. The Food and Drug Administration constantly attempts to remind the public of the overdose danger of OTC drugs. Yet despite these warnings, the agency found, "the public does not regard these products (OTC drugs) as medicine which, if used improperly, can cause injury or death."

In normal doses, the trivial side effects of aspirin are common, while the serious ones are extremely rare. The most common trivial side effect is undetectable without special medical examination. About two-thirds of all persons who take normal aspirin doses bleed an insignificant extra half-teaspoon of blood through their stomachs, compared with the normal half-teaspoon they lose daily without having taken any aspirin. (Shaving and toothbrushing, among other common activities, result also in comparable loss of blood.)

The most common detectable side effect of aspirin is stomach upset, either nausea or heartburn, which affects perhaps 2,000 out of 100,000 persons who take aspirin. Compare that to the frequency of the most serious side effect at normal doses: an asthma-like allergic reaction occurs in about 4 persons out of 100,000 in the general population. Harmful stomach bleeding or ulcers, which *may* be related to aspirin use, are found in 25 out of 100,000 persons who take aspirin regularly.

Adding up overlapping side effects overstates the case. Leaving out insignificant internal bleeding and excluding imagined stomach upset, only 5 percent of the population could suffer side effects from normal aspirin doses, while 95 percent would not.

Large or frequent aspirin doses cause side effects more frequently. The Boston Collaborative Drug Surveillance Program (BCDSP) examined the hospital records of 2,391 persons taking aspirin and found total side effects, major and minor, in 5 percent of the patients. Single doses of three or more tablets were eight times as likely to cause side effects as two-tablet doses. A daily dosage of more than nine tablets was forty-three times more likely to cause side effects than a daily dose of four tablets or less.

Normal Dose Reactions

Aspirin is a weak acid; like most other acids, it upsets the gastrointestinal system, which maintains a balance between acids and base substances, creating chemicals to counter those ingested. When the balance is upset, the system corrects it, usually before adverse effects occur.

The operation of the gastrointestinal system explains the time and dose dependency of aspirin side effects. Ten tablets taken at once overwhelm the acid-base balance in most people; side effects result until the balance is righted. Spreading the ten tablets out during a day would produce less drastic change in acid content, allowing the system to balance one batch of aspirin's acid before the next was ingested.

Minor stomach upset is an occasional result of the acid imbalance caused by aspirin. The imbalance can even result in nausea, if the patient already has an upset or empty stomach. When acid splashes into the throat from the stomach, the result is heartburn. Both upset and heartburn usually disappear within hours, as the aspirin's acid is neutralized.

Stomach Bleeding

Stomach bleeding from normal doses of aspirin, while common, is medically insignificant. Aspirin causes bleeding because it is an acid and because it decreases platelet stickiness. Although the stomach normally contains its own acid to aid digestion, extra acid, such as aspirin, if it adheres to the stomach wall at one spot, can irritate, causing microscopic patches of stomach lining to flake off.

Whether lining disturbances precede or follow an aspirin dose, they will bleed slightly longer in the presence of aspirin. Since lining breaks are very small injuries, their bleeding would normally be blocked by platelets until a clot could form. Aspirin reduces platelets' ability to plug very small injuries.

Philosophically, concern over stomach bleeding may be shrugged off with the logic of Dr. Mervyn Sahud, a blood specialist who testified before an FDA panel in 1972. He said, "Whatever increased blood loss might be attributed to the presence of the aspirin effect on platelets is simply insignificant when compared to the therapeutic benefit of the product."

Physically, aspirin-caused stomach bleeding was discounted as a major effect in a 1972 study conducted by Dr. Ivan Danhof of the University of Texas. He examined 100 persons between the ages of twenty-one and sixty-two to determine their normal stomach blood loss and their loss after taking aspirin.

He examined the subjects for four days and found 95 percent lost one-half teaspoon or less of blood through their stomach daily, when their eating habits were normal.

Danhof then gave ten subjects twelve aspirin tablets daily for twelve days. While taking aspirin, their blood loss increased to about a teaspoon a day. Medically, the amount had "absolutely no significance," Danhof reported, even over a long period of time. When doses were continued for longer periods, the loss decreased but did not drop to normal.

For comparison, Danhof examined the blood loss caused by a spicy Mexican meal. Subjects ate a normal breakfast, then ate a lunch and dinner of spicy Mexican food in the laboratory. Two tablespoons of jalapeño pepper hot sauce were required at each Mexican meal. The amount of sauce used would figuratively "set anyone's innards on fire," Danhof said lightly.

Overall, the spicy meals caused only about one-third as much bleeding as aspirin. However, Danhof found some subjects were sensitive to hot sauce; they lost as much blood from the spicy meals as most people lost after taking aspirin.

Danhof concluded that aspirin-caused blood loss was statistically detectable after ingestion of twelve aspirin tablets per day. "But I feel that the amount of blood loss for the average patient is well within the limit for him to compensate for his loss. This is particularly true considering that when the doses are continued, there is an apparent tolerance—so with subsequent treatment days, there is a decrease in the amount of blood loss."

The Boston Collaborative Drug Surveillance Program found persons admitted to the hospital with serious stomach bleeding were twice as likely to be regular aspirin takers as similar patients without bleeding. The BCDSP found about 13 persons out of 100,000 in the general population are admitted to the hospital each year for stomach bleeding; among those taking aspirin four times a week, the figure is 28, an increase of 15 per 100,000, which may be attributable to aspirin. It may also be that regular aspirin users have other habit or lifestyle patterns that make them more prone to stomach bleeding.

Ulcers

There are two major ulcer locations, the stomach and the intestines. Peptic ulcers are a loss of lining in either area; gastric ulcers are a loss of stomach lining, while duodenal ulcers are a loss of intestine lining. When the lining is lost, normal gastric acid reacts with the underlying tissue, causing pain, bleeding, or both.

Aspirin has been weakly associated with peptic ulcers and most weakly associated with gastric ulcers. Physically, aspirin disturbs the stomach and intestinal lining and may increase lining damage by reducing prostaglandin (PG) production.

PG's apparently protect the intestinal tract from its own acid, either by protecting the lining or aiding in its healing once breached. Scientists have found more PG's in the stomachs of persons without ulcers than are present in persons with ulcers. In one experiment, 42 percent of the ulcers in a PG-treated group were healed after two weeks, compared to 14 percent in a similar untreated group. Whether PG's protect or heal, a decreased PG level caused by aspirin could explain aspirin's contribution to ulceration.

A BCDSP study found persons who took aspirin four times a week were more likely to be entering the hospital because of a new, non-cancerous stomach ulcer than those who took aspirin less often. The researchers found taking aspirin could be responsible for a hospital admission rate for ulcers in 13 persons out of 100,000 each year, compared with 3 per 100,000 in the general population, an increase of 10 per 100,000.

The BCDSP could not rule out the chance that the higher admission rate for aspirin-takers was the result of doctors searching for signs of an ulcer more carefully among such patients. This could increase the reported frequency of ulcer admissions among heavy aspirin users.

The overall risk of either condition is slight, in terms of public-health risks. Ulcers and stomach bleeding resulting in hospitalization are increased jointly by 25 out of 100,000 persons per year among heavy aspirin users. Yet the public has apparently decided the risk of birth-control pills is acceptable, and they result in 60 admissions for clot treatment among 100,000 users each year (there is no known indication or contraindication for aspirin taking among women on the pill).

Aspirin Intolerance

The rare problem of aspirin intolerance, or idiosyncracy, at normal doses is not significant: it is rarely fatal in the first attack and most persons avoid aspirin once the idiosyncracy has manifested itself.

Aspirin idiosyncracy causes hives, asthma-like attacks, a swollen face, tongue, or lips, and sometimes blocks breathing. Such symptoms usually occur immediately after aspirin is taken. Other symptoms include coughing, wheezing, a tight feeling in the chest, and, very rarely, unconsciousness or death.

The condition can suddenly manifest itself during a person's twenties or thirties, even if they have never had previous symptoms. Such was the case with Lt. Commander John S. Bull, an astronaut, who was thirty-three before he first showed signs of aspirin idiosyncracy. A Navy flyer, he was dropped from the NASA program in 1968 because of his condition. His case began in November, 1967, with sinus problems. Later that winter, he caught a persistent cough, then had an asthma-like attack in January, 1968.

Aspirin idiosyncracy is observed most commonly among asthmatics, who comprise 4 percent of the U.S. population. Idiosyncracy's overall incidence is about 4 persons out of 100,000 in the general population.

Abnormal Dose Reactions

When taken more than three tablets at once or more often than every four hours, aspirin sometimes causes life-threatening side effects. The amount of aspirin and the time between doses needed to cause such effects vary with body chemistry and weight.

As mentioned before, however, it must be noted that *all* drugs, taken too often or in oversize doses, pose serious health hazards. Although non-prescription or over-the-counter drugs are frequently thought of as hazard-free, they can be just as dangerous as more powerful prescription drugs if they are abused. The following catalogue of aspirin effects in overdose should not be construed as a recommendation against aspirin; a listing of the side effects or any substitute, including acetaminophen, would be just as long and frightening. In fact, as mentioned before, some physicians find acetaminophen poisoning more insidious than aspirin poisoning, since it is harder to reverse and may take seventy-two hours to exhibit its symptoms.

Overdoses of aspirin are called salicylism (after the name of aspirin's chemical family) or aspirin poisoning, and are typified by a series of increasingly serious central nervous system disruptions.

The earliest symptom of salicylism that the victim can detect is ringing ears, followed at progressively larger doses by deafness. Such deafness is usually of short duration and its severity is dose-dependent. This warning sign comes well before more serious side effects and has convinced physicians that accidental overdose is unlikely among adults; they believe most aspirin poisoning is intentionally self-inflicted.

In a BCDSP study, aspirin-caused deafness occurred among 1 percent of all aspirin-takers, and in clear relationship to their doses. Deafness struck 11 percent of those taking three or more aspirin at once, compared with .06 percent of those taking a more normal one or two-tablet dose. The deafness studied ended when the aspirin dose was cut or halted.

Acid-base imbalance and central nervous system disruption are the major symptoms of more serious salicylism, caused by toxic doses of aspirin. The imbalance makes a person's breath smell like acetone, or nail-polish remover; similar, in that sense, to a severe diabetic attack. After an aspirin overdose, the kidneys, which remove poisons from the blood, are overwhelmed; as a result, nearly every other organ is adversely affected by circulating toxins.

The nerves that control automatic breathing are disrupted by poisonous aspirin doses: breathing either stops, or becomes so slow and sporadic that a dangerous build-up of carbon dioxide occurs, encouraging formation of more acid and further disturbing the acid-base balance.

Vomiting, dizziness, headaches, confusion, depression, and delirium can result from disruption of the central nervous system by salicylism. Excess carbon dioxide in the blood can cause convulsions and unconsciousness.

Aspirin and Children

Since the amount of aspirin needed to cause salicylism is proportional to body weight, children are especially vulnerable to overdoses. According to the AMA *Drug Evaluations,* the most common form of fatal drug poisoning in children is aspirin poisoning.

The federal government recognized the danger aspirin poses to children when Congress passed the 1970 Poison Prevention Packaging Act. Under the act, the first four substances required to be placed in child-proof containers were prescription drugs, furniture polish, drain cleaner, and aspirin.

The largest known dose of aspirin survived by a minor was 50 tablets, comparable to the maximum survivable adult dose of approximately 100 tablets. Adults can be killed by as few as 12 tablets if they are unusually sensitive; very young children can be killed by a single adult tablet.

About 65,000 children are admitted to hospitals each year suffering from aspirin poisoning, but only a very small percentage die, according to John Mennear, professor of toxicology at Purdue University in Lafayette, Indiana. He attributes the low rate to awareness of the aspirin-poisoning problem and the fact that rapid treatment nearly always prevents death.

Home first aid for aspirin overdose is simple and should be begun immediately for either child or adult, simultaneously with a call to the family physician, the local poison-control center or the nearest hospital emergency room. It is important to know which aspirin product has been taken, the weight and age of the patient and approximately how many aspirin tablets were involved. With these facts, medical personnel can advise whether or not a trip to the hospital is necessary.

The first aid should begin by inducing vomiting, using an ounce of Ipacac or some other means. Then, give the patient milk, fruit juice, or charcoal to delay abosorption of the aspirin remaining in the system.

In severe cases, where the patient is unconscious or in convulsions, begin artificial respiration immediately and take him or her to the hospital without calling. Bring along the aspirin bottle.

The two best means of preventing aspirin overdose in children are to keep aspirin out of their reach and to avoid designating aspirin (or any other drug) as "candy" in order to encourage a child to take it.

Aspirin poisoning is remarkably rare, considering its universal availability and the small amounts needed to poison children under five, who comprise 70 percent of the childhood poisoning victims.

Non-Effects

Some members of the general public mistakenly believe aspirin causes birth defects. One Australian study, of women who took two to twelve aspirin tablets a day during pregnancy, suggested a possibly increased incidence of birth defects. But the study was not supported by a later study of aspirin and birth defects among 50,282 women in 12 U.S. hospitals. Aspirin-taking during the first four months of pregnancy, when defects are believed created, was studied. Researchers found 35,418 women said they had taken no aspirin; 9,736 some; and 5,128 said they took aspirin more than 8 days a month.

The study found the statistically expected number of birth defects, no matter what the aspirin-taking level.

An FDA advisory panel has recommended that pregnant women not take aspirin during the last three months of pregnancy, but this was not based on a fear of birth defects. Rather, it is intended to avoid aspirin's effect of increasing bleeding time, which can make complicated deliveries more difficult.

There are also members of the public who believe aspirin impairs kidney function. There were reports in the 1960s linking phenacetin to kidney damage: in such products as APC, Empirin, and others, phenacetin is mixed with aspirin. The BCDSP examined the records of 6,407 hospital patients and found no significant relationship between aspirin-taking and impaired kidney function.

On Balance

The preponderance of evidence on aspirin risks and benefits is clearly in favor of its known benefits. A 1974 *New England Journal of Medicine* editorial stated the same conclusion. It said withholding aspirin without better cause than "fear of stomach problems" was "extremely questionable" for "a patient who desperately requires the relief provided by this excellent analgesic."

That is the state of the risk-benefit ratio today. The ratio could improve even more if aspirin were found to have an important new benefit; the ability to reduce heart-attack risk. It very well may, as discussed in the next chapter.

7

Aspirin and Cardiovascular Disease

Half of all deaths after middle age result from cardiovascular (CV) diseases; that is, diseases of the heart and blood vessels, including heart attacks, strokes, and related conditions. CV diseases often cause rapid death, allowing little time for treatment. Many patients who survive a first attack find it difficult to change their habits in order to avoid recurrence; it is not always easy to lose weight, avoid certain foods, or give up cigarettes and get more exercise.

So, physicians seeking to prolong life are looking for a drug with virtually no side effects, which reduces the risk of these diseases among those who have had neither symptoms nor an attack—because often, the first symptom is death. Alternatively, they seek a drug with reasonable side effects, for use by persons who have experienced one attack, because their odds of a second attack are greatly increased.

It is difficult to imagine a drug that has a low risk to benefit ratio for a symptom-free, attack-free person. Even the slightest risk from a drug used to "pretreat" such persons might be more significant than the CV disease risk of the symptomless. But the risk of a second heart attack is five times greater than the first attack risk of the general public. Likewise, a "little stroke" victim is much more likely to have a real stroke than a person who has never had an attack. So, a small risk of side effects would be much more acceptable among the at-risk population of those who have had one heart attack or "little stroke."

At the present time, no drug seems likely to be so risk-free that persons with no symptoms and no attack history should take it *en masse* to avoid a first attack or stroke. However, some physicians believe there is a drug whose side effects are sufficiently rare that it could be recommended to those who have had one attack or have a high-risk lifestyle: aspirin.

Aspirin's action as an anti-platelet drug has become well understood only in recent years. This action now offers a theoretical basis for the observed possibility that aspirin reduces the risk of heart attacks. After more than three-quarters of a century of worldwide usage, aspirin's side effects are known to be infrequent. But before there can be a universal prescription of aspirin to reduce heart-attack risk, a link must be forged between laboratory theory and practical effect, by testing on large numbers of persons leading normal lives.

The significance of a drug that substantially reduces the toll of CV diseases is difficult to imagine. Like arthritis, CV diseases are chronic; incurable, their control requires years of treatment. Yet the lifestyle changes now required of those suffering from CV disease are even more difficult than those required of arthritics— many of whom can lead nearly normal lives, thanks in part to control of their disease by aspirin.

Aspirin now appears to hold the bright promise of similar control for heart-attack and stroke victims. Some encouraging studies have been completed, others are underway. Most theoretical and experimental data points to a new role for aspirin in controlling an impressive portion of modern man's cardiovascular diseases.

Clotting and Blood

Aspirin's effect on CV-disease risk derives from its effect on clotting, the mechanism of chemicals and cells that protects the circulatory system from loss of blood when operating normally—but can cause death from lack of blood flow when operating abnormally.

When it is working properly, the clotting process is set in motion by a cut or rupture in a blood vessel. The system plugs the hole and aids the growth of new vessel wall at the injury site. When the process is not functioning properly, it forms unneeded and dangerous clots, which can block seemingly healthy blood vessels.

The clotting process protects both parts of the bloodstream: bright red blood, under high pressure in arteries, carrying nutrients and oxygen to cells; darker blood under low pressure in veins, carrying carbon dioxide and waste. The body's disease defenses are carried in the blood, as are clotting-system components.

Plasma is the liquid that carries the blood, consisting of 94.2 percent red cells (carrying gas, food, and waste), .2 percent white cells (defending against disease) and 5.6 percent platelets (aiding clotting). The platelet, a colorless disc one-third the size of a red cell, is the simplest blood cell; the body's entire platelet supply is renewed every nine to twelve days, so an average cell is replaced in about five days.

When a vessel is injured, clotting begins within seconds: the vessel wall contracts and platelets start forming a temporary plug. Within minutes a stronger, more permanent fibrin clot is formed on top of the platelet plug. In either hours or days (depending on the size of the injury) the fibrin clot is dissolved and replaced with new vessel wall tissue.

The differences between arteries and veins lead to different clotting patterns in the two halves of the bloodstream. Platelet plugs predominate in the high-pressure, high-volume arteries because attempts to build stronger fibrin clots are usually washed away quickly. In the veins, however, the slow-moving blood will not wash away fibrin clots, which can form on the slightest injury.

CV Diseases

Clots are not the cause of cardiovascular disease, but they are a major contributing factor. The mechanism of clot formation in injured vessels and arteries is known; the trigger of clot formation in seemingly uninjured vessels is still in question. Excess weight, smoking, and a lack of exercise, as well as certain dietary habits, are believed to contribute to the formation of clots in uninjured blood vessels.

Whatever their cause, CV diseases take a significant toll: they cause half the natural deaths in the United States each year. Cardiovascular-disease deaths cost the nation $22.7 billion each year in lost services, according to the American Heart Association. Similar statistics apply throughout the technologically developed countries.

Although CV diseases can and do appear in persons of any age, they are typically diseases of the elderly. Heart attacks are rare among persons below age forty; strokes are uncommon among persons under the age of sixty.

One CV disease, thromboembolism, occurs when a blood clot forms and breaks off into the bloodstream. The condition seldom occurs naturally, but is the most common cause of death after surgery. About 100,000 persons die and 300,000 are hospitalized each year in the United States as a result of thromboembolism.

Another CV disease, "little strokes," occurs when the arteries supplying blood to the brain are blocked for a few seconds. The condition is also known as a "transient ischemic attack" (TIA). If the arteries are blocked longer, a full stroke results, usually causing some degree of permanent damage to brain cells. Half the 200,000 strokes in the United States each year are fatal. A cumulative total of 200,000 stroke survivors were "aphasic" as of 1976; unable to either read and write or speak and hear normally. Many other survivors have lesser physical or mental handicaps as the result of their strokes.

Venous Clots

Thromboembolism is primarily a disorder of the veins, the low-pressure system. Venous clots usually form in the legs, often as the result of prolonged pressure and lack of movement, such as from lying in bed after surgery. No sign of irregularity or break in the blood vessel wall is usually found near the clot. Venous clots are sometimes disease-related, as in phlebitis, a disease which afflicted former President Richard Nixon.

When venous clots grow, they can cause pain, tenderness and swelling. If such clots grow large enough, they threaten the blood supply to tissue.

More often, as was the case with Nixon, the greater danger of a venous clot comes when it breaks away from the point of formation and travels through the bloodstream. Then it becomes a thromboembolus, literally a traveling clot. If the venous clot then enters the lungs and blocks blood flow, death often results. If the venous clot crosses over into the arteries it can induce a heart attack or stroke in the same fashion as an arterial plug or clot.

Arterial Clots

Heart attack and stroke are the major CV diseases involving disturbance of the arterial blood vessels, in which blood moves away from the heart under high pressure.

Heart attacks, the often-fatal death of all or part of the heart muscle, are known by several medical terms which specify their cause. The most general term is myocardial infarction, which means death of heart tissue, from whatever cause.

Disease and valve defects present since birth or induced by injury are the major non-clot causes of heart attacks. But they cause an insignificant number of attacks compared with clot-induced irregular heartbeat or blocked and hardened arteries.

Full strokes involve the death of brain tissue caused by decreased or halted blood supply. Tumors or blood loss from broken or leaky arteries (cerebral hemorrhage) may cause strokes. But clot-related blockages are a more common cause.

"Little strokes" stem from the same causes, but often serve only as precursors to a full stroke. Untold thousands of persons suffer from them each year. They cause blindness or paralysis for periods of time ranging from a few seconds to several hours. Although they sometimes cause permanent damage, "little strokes" more often have a beneficial purpose—to serve as a warning signal.

A medical journal advertisement describes a "little stroke:" "My left arm and leg went out of control, kind of, and I couldn't make them work right. My coordination was terrible. I'd reach for a glass of water and knock it over. I sat down for a few minutes and then I was OK."

Atherosclerosis

Atherosclerosis, also known as hardening of the arteries, is an arterial, clot-related condition and a major cause of CV diseases. Arterial clots, usually no more than platelet plugs, may trigger the atherosclerotic process; they certainly contribute to its development.

By itself, atherosclerosis can gradually narrow veins and arteries and slowly kill the heart or brain tissue with a reduced blood supply. Together with clots, atherosclerosis can cause sudden death. Clots large enough to block open blood vessels are rare; clots large enough to block hardened arteries are more common.

The trigger that initiates hardening of the arteries is unknown, but platelets are likely suspects. In a healthy blood vessel, platelets can stick to a virus, bacteria, or chemical compound. Once a few platelets stick, they release chemicals that make other platelets stick to them and that allow a mass of platelets to stick to a healthy vessel wall, making it irregular.

Once the wall is irregular, whether because of platelets or some other trigger, the atherosclerotic process begins. Platelets play a role in the process, as do several other factors.

Platelets will stick to an irregular blood vessel surface and form an incipient plug. If arterial pressure does not wash it away, the plug will grow and stimulate the surrounding vessel wall.

The blood vessel will grow to cover the plug, using cholesterol and other chemicals as building blocks to narrow the vessel. The surface of the new section is often irregular, attracting more platelets and starting the process over again.

Layers of new blood vessel wall, alternating between platelet plugs and new cell walls like an onion skin, progressively narrow the artery. This process primarily affects the vessels supplying blood to the brain and heart.

Atherosclerosis plays a role in almost all heart attacks and strokes. Attacks of these two CV diseases can be divided into two classes: attacks that kill within minutes and attacks that kill more than a day after the first symptoms.

Hardened arteries are found in autopsies after most heart attacks and strokes that do not result in immediate death. The attacks are gradual, rather than sudden, and the first symptoms really indicate the endpoint of a long-term process of tissue death caused by decreased blood flow.

Sudden tissue death, caused by a complete cutoff of blood supply, may result in a patient's death within minutes of first suffering pain. These attacks result when an artery, narrowed by atherosclerosis, is blocked by a clot. Such attacks are specifically called coronary thrombosis (blocked heart artery) and cerebral thrombosis (blocked brain artery); once believed to be the major source of heart attacks and strokes, these conditions are now known to be rare.

Clots can also cause sudden attacks without blocking an artery. In the heart, clots irritate the internal pacemaker, causing fatal irregularities in the heartbeat. In the brain, clots irritate blood vessels, causing a sudden constriction that can block a vessel many times their size. Because of the critical nature of brain blood flow, vessels there are more sensitive than elsewhere in the body.

Non-Drug Clot Control

Doctors have a number of means, besides drugs, to minimize formation of clots in blood vessels, thereby decreasing the incidence of cardiovascular episodes. Perhaps the riskiest is surgical clot removal. Besides the risks common to all surgery, clot removal runs the special risk of dislodging the clot, so that it moves to another narrowed vessel and quite possibly causes rapid death. Also, the areas in which many clots form are nearly inaccessible to the surgeon.

Two surgical techniques have proven to be among the success-ful non-drug methods of cardiovascular disease control through reduction of clot formation. Platelets are most likely to gather in blood vessels with fatty deposits in them, and these platelet aggre-gations commonly trigger strokes. The most accessible site of such deposits is the carotid artery in the neck, which is cut open, cleaned and sewn shut in an often successful effort to cut stroke risk.

The similar surgical procedure for reduction of clotting risk near the heart is coronary bypass surgery, in which fat-clogged arteries near the heart are bypassed entirely by new blood vessels brought from elsewhere in the body.

Physical therapy is used to prevent the formation of both ven-ous and arterial clots, and to reduce the risk of their blocking a ves-sel. Venous clots, frequently the result of lack of blood movement, are combatted by elevating patients' legs, to keep blood moving out of them and reduce the chance of clot formation on slight stimuli.

For arterial clots, physical treatment is much different. Plate-let plugs have obviously already been formed, despite the rapid movement of blood in the arteries, if a person has had a heart at-tack or stroke. So the initial treatment in these cases is to reduce movement, to minimize the chance of further clots breaking off from their source.

Persons who recover from heart attacks, generally those at-tacks caused by reduced flow in hardened arteries, are encouraged to minimize the possible effect of future clots through exercise. Faster blood flow discourages platelet formation; it also builds up alternative blood supplies in the heart, reducing the effect of future artery-blocking clots.

Lifestyle changes are often recommended to reduce clotting risk among patients who have shown a tendency to form clots, either through chemical tests or by an actual attack. Weight loss and cessation of smoking are often suggested. In addition to the lung damage caused by smoking, some researchers believe nicotine from cigarette smoke increases the rate at which the body replaces platelets. Young platelets are stickier than old platelets and are more likely to form clots. Reduced weight can lower the heart's working burden, making it less likely to fail if small parts die from lack of blood.

A controversial change is diet. Some doctors recommend diets high in unsaturated fats, such as vegetable oil, and low in saturated fats, such as animal fat and dairy products. This is intended to reduce the blood level of cholestorol, a building block of atherosclerosis. Other doctors think dietary cholestorol controls are worthless; they say the liver will manufacture the chemical if it is missing from the diet. Researchers have recently found there are two types of cholesterol: one may build up fat, the other may decrease fat.

Clot Control with Drugs

There are three major classes of drugs used to control clots: thrombolytic (which break up clots), anti-coagulant (which reduce or prevent fibrin clots) and anti-platelet drugs (which prevent formation of platelet plugs). Each entails a degree of risk; at the present time, these drugs are not used to prevent first attacks, only to control recurrence or when tests indicate a high-risk blood condition.

The thrombolytic drugs are most useful in reducing the size of recent, venous clots. Their side effects are numerous, however, so their use is generally restricted to young, previously healthy patients. Their disadvantages include possible immune reaction and expense. Persons with ulcers, asthma, or high blood pressure cannot generally be given these drugs.

There are more than 100 anti-coagulant drugs, all of which minimize fibrin clot formation. Their use requires close medical supervision in order to prevent severe bleeding as a side effect. Traditionally, these drugs have been given to heart-attack and stroke victims to reduce the high risk of recurrence. However, platelet plugs are the primary triggering agents of these two diseases, not the fibrin clots prevented by anti-coagulants.

Anti-coagulants are useful in some attack victims; they reduce by half the 6 percent chance of death from venous, fibrin clot complications after a first heart attack or stroke. But the vast majority of persons who survive die from a recurrence which usually involves arterial platelet plugs. Anti-coagulant therapy does not appear to be the most promising method of treatment for them.

Anti-platelet drugs, among them aspirin, interfere with the platelets' tendency to stick to each other and to a wound or irritation; these drugs make platelets demonstrably less sticky. Since platelets are believed to start atherosclerosis and are known to contribute to its development, their control is an important part of efforts to fight this disease. Regardless of their role in atherosclerosis, platelets are the primary component of death-dealing clots moving through the arteries.

Aspirin and Platelets

Platelet plugs play a key role in CV disease; prostaglandins play a key role in platelet plug formation. Anti-platelet drugs, which interfere with prostaglandin (PG) production, are an important part of the drug arsenal used to fight CV disease.

As mentioned before, platelets stick to irregular surfaces and breaks on blood vessel walls. Only the few platelets that actually contact the irregularity stick by direct action. The majority of a platelet plug is formed by platelet-platelet sticking. This sticking is caused by released chemicals, foremost among them, PGs. One type of PG makes vessel walls constrict; another makes platelet-platelet sticking easier.

Platelets attracted to a large wound release so many other chemicals that PGs are not required to cause sticking. But an irregularity, as opposed to a wound, may attract so few platelets that, in the absence of PGs, no plug forms. Irregularities are more likely to be atherosclerotic surfaces than wounds requiring plugs, so failure of plugs to form on them is a positive, rather than a negative, event.

98

When two aspirin are ingested, virtually all the platelets in the body are "acetylated" by the products aspirin releases in the bloodstream. Acetylation renders inoperative the enzyme in the platelet that manufactures PGs. An acetylated platelet will make no more PGs until it is replaced. The body takes ten days to replace its entire platelet supply, so daily aspirin usage keeps 90 percent of a person's platelets acetylated at all times.

As a result, daily aspirin ingestion, in theory, could prevent platelet plugs from forming, except on wounds or gross blood vessel irregularities. This theory has been tested successfully in laboratories and on animals, but clinical tests on humans are needed to determine aspirin's effect on cardiovascular disease.

Aspirin Studies

Although aspirin's effect on platelets was not discovered until 1967, its apparent effect on heart attack and stroke was reported in 1956. This early report was greeted with a great deal of skepticism.

Dr. Lawrence L. Craven was a general practitioner in Glendale, California. After forty years of practice, he decided to limit himself to the treatment of older patients. Since many persons in the older age group suffered heart attacks and strokes, he wrote, he became "interested in the possibility that some simple harmless agent may be effective against the two major causes of death and disability among the persons who have the most to contribute to our civilization."

In the late 1940s, anti-coagulant therapy had been introduced to prevent recurrence of heart attack and stroke. Craven noted such drug use was unsuitable for large numbers of persons because of the need for constant monitoring of dose and effect. He also scoffed at treatment after the first attack in general, since it required that physicians "waited until after the initial damage had been done and then attempted to prevent further damage."

In 1950, Craven published a brief paper describing his intention to study the effects of aspirin. In the September, 1956, issue of the same journal, the obscure *Mississippi Valley Medical Journal*, he announced a "simple but surprisingly effective means" of preventing second heart attacks and possibly even first ones; taking one or two aspirin tablets a day.

Aspirin appeared harmless in most instances and could be life-saving, since it was known to increase bleeding time, Dr. Craven reasoned. (It would take another eleven years for researchers to find out exactly why aspirin increased bleeding time.) He began taking aspirin himself and recommended it to his friends and patients. The results were printed in bold type in the 1956 article: "Not a single case of detectable coronary or cerebral thrombosis has occurred" among 8,000 patients following the aspirin regimen for as long as ten years.

He described the participants as healthy, but also as obese and infrequent exercisers, making them "tailored for heart attacks."

Dr. Craven did not say how many patients died, or of what causes. He said nine apparent heart-attack deaths proved, after examination, to result from other causes. He said there were minor strokes, but no major ones, yet again provided no figures.

Dr. Craven was not disturbed because he could not be certain how aspirin worked to prevent CV disease. The important result, to him, was living patients: "To any physician who has witnessed the results of long-term aspirin administration—who has seen his patients freed of their fear of heart attacks at a time when their contemporaries are stricken down with coronary and cerebral thrombosis, the evidence speaks for itself."

There are a number of grounds on which Craven's study could be attacked. Some critics pointed out that he assumed aspirin was an anti-coagulant without any medical proof. Others called attention to the fact that his study was not controlled, that is, he did not compare the group regularly taking aspirin with a similar non-aspirin-taking group. Since Craven ran the study and examined all the patients himself, and had decided in advance what he wanted to find, his reports could hardly be described as unbiased. His study made no reference to checks on whether his patients complied with his aspirin regimen, and contains no comment on side effects, except to note that aspirin taking "certainly carries no hazard. However, it may be lifesaving."

As with the Rev. Edmund Stone's observations of the use of willow bark for fever, which led to the discovery of salicylic acid and later aspirin, Craven's study would win low marks for scientific validity but high marks for well-intentioned observation. Other, more careful observers, would provide a more reliable basis for reaching the same conclusion: aspirin may substantially reduce the risk of heart attack and stroke.

Thromboembolism Studies

Drugs that might be used as preventative treatments for clot formation are widely studied by those trying to prevent thromboembolism, clots moving in the bloodstream.

The need for prevention, rather than treatment, was vividly outlined in 1976, by Boston bone specialists Dr. William Harris and Dr. Edwin Salzman. In the *Journal of Joint and Bone Surgery* they pointed out that when clots travel to the lung, death occurs within thirty minutes in two-thirds of all patients, much too fast for after-the-fact therapy. Finding clots before they break off is difficult and the tests are unreliable, they wrote, so pre-treatment cannot be limited to only the highest-risk patients. If there is reasonable risk, Harris and Salzman concluded, safe and effective drug therapy is called for.

According to two studies, both published in 1976, one possibly safe and effective drug for prevention of clots is aspirin. Both studies examined postoperative clots, those that most commonly lead to thromboembolism.

In Fitzroy, Australia, 160 patients over age forty at St. Vincent's Hospital were randomly divided into groups of 75 and 85. The two groups were similar in major characteristics, and entered the hospital for elective surgery. The control group was untreated after the operation; the other group was given aspirin and another drug.

Only 14 percent of the aspirin group developed clots, compared to 28 percent of the untreated group. No complications were reported in the aspirin group. Although the other drug had a more powerful anti-platelet effect, taking it with aspirin allowed a lower dose and decreased its incidence of side effects. The report concluded the two drugs showed promise as a preventative treatment for clot formation after operations.

In a Boston study, 528 hospital patients were given two aspirin tablets twice a day prior to hip replacement surgery. The high risk of clots in such cases caused researchers to avoid using an untreated control group, so the results were open to some question. Normally, there would be 10 fatal lung clots and 53 non-fatal lung clots in a group of 528 patients. The treated group suffered no fatal clots and only seven non-fatal ones. The researchers concluded, "Aspirin may be a simple and useful" preventative agent in hip surgery.

Prospective and Retrospective

The studies detailed in the remainder of this chapter fall into two categories, prospective and retrospective. The difference between the two categories is subtle. A retrospective study examines actions already taken that were not directly observed, usually through interview information. A prospective study is one in which actions are examined as they occur.

A retrospective study might involve asking stroke victims and other persons in the same age group about their aspirin-taking habits, then concluding those who suffer strokes are less likely to have taken aspirin. A prospective study of the same question would match an aspirin-taking group against an identical non-aspirin-taking group. Its conclusion might be that those who take aspirin are less likely to have strokes. The difference between the two statements is subtle, but apparent upon examination. Retrospective studies are considered useful as indicators, but are generally regarded as insufficent without subsequent studies.

Stroke Studies

"I think it is interesting to note that aspirin, which has been used extensively for treating minor headaches, is now being considered as prophylaxis (pretreatment) against headaches of a more serious nature (strokes)," said Columbia University blood specialist Dr. Harvey Weiss in 1971.

Before aspirin can be used as a stroke preventative, its effects must be tested in people. Several such tests, retrospective and prospective, have been conducted. Completed tests indicate aspirin may be useful.

In a 1974 retrospective study, researchers at the Indiana University School of Medicine examined the medical histories of fifteen aspirin-treated subjects and eleven non-treated subjects. All had suffered "little strokes." There were nine further attacks in the untreated group and two in the treated group; otherwise the groups were the same. The standard aspirin dose was two tablets a day—but the two treated patients with recurrent attacks had no further attacks when their dose was doubled.

The results of an interesting prospective study were published in 1977. Sponsored by the National Heart, Lung and Blood Institute (NHLBI, an agency of the federal department of Health, Education, and Welfare), doctors at ten university-related hospitals around the United States reported to University of Texas researchers on the effects of regular aspirin taking on "little strokes".

There were 179 stroke patients in the study, average age sixty, randomly assigned to a control group or a treated group. The treated group got two aspirin tablets daily; the control group received identical placebos. Neither doctor nor patient knew to which group a patient was assigned.

Dr. William S. Fields reported no statistically significant difference between the groups, if the patient had only one attack within three months of entering the program, although aspirin slightly reduced attack recurrence and death even in this group.

But among patients suffering multiple attacks in the three

months prior to entering the program, 87.5 percent of the treated group was free of unfavorable symptoms, while only 58.5 percent of the control group was symptom-free. Included among "unfavorable" symptoms were death, stroke, and increased numbers of "little strokes."

Conclusive evidence of aspirin's effect on stroke risk may be forthcoming from the Canadian Cooperative Study of Recurrent Presumed Cerebral Emboli, also known as the Canadian Cooperative Study. Patients were still being registered for the program during 1977. Once 550 patients have been selected, the test will run five years, comparing the effects of aspirin to other drugs and to a placebo. Physicians and statisticians at McMaster University in Hamilton, Ontario, are coordinating doctors at twelve centers in six provinces who are performing the study. At an October 1978 meeting in West Berlin, a leader of the Canadian study reported that their statisticians had broken the code of the double-blind study and determined that aspirin reduced TIAs, completed strokes and death from stroke by 50 percent in males. No such effect was noted in female subjects in the investigation. The reason for this marked difference in response between the sexes was not clear.

Heart-Attack Studies

Aspirin has been widely studied for its usefulness in preventing heart attacks; but completed studies were not conclusive. They indicated, but did not prove, that aspirin may reduce the risk of heart attacks. The only researcher ever to claim 100 percent effectiveness was Craven, whose methods have been called into doubt. But even if aspirin reduces heart-attack risk 50 percent, it will be a major breakthrough, proving to be faster, less expensive, and easier than other prevention methods.

The major retrospective study of aspirin-taking and heart attacks was conducted in 1974 by the Boston Collaborative Drug Surveillance Program. The number of patients involved and the statistical significance of the difference between aspirin-takers and non-takers makes the study particularly interesting.

Since 1966, the BCDSP has been the only large-scale program measuring the effects of all drugs, including aspirin, on hospital patients. Trained nurses serve as monitors in the program, recording drug use prior to and during hospitalization. They also note side effects, doctors' determinations of effectiveness and diagnosis when a patient is discharged. The information is then placed on computer tapes for analysis. Information has been collected on about 60,000 patients during the program's first eleven years.

There were two parts to the 1974 BCDSP heart attack study. One used regular BCDSP data, which contained no extra information for the purpose of studying heart-attack risk. The other part of the study involved asking patients extra questions about pre-hospitalization drug use and heart-attack risk factors. Persons above sixty-nine and below forty were excluded from both studies. Groups of aspirin-takers and non-takers were selected to be similar in terms of important characteristics.

In the first part of the study, using regular data on 8,154 patients, those who took aspirin regularly within six weeks of admission were one-fifth as likely to have been admitted for a heart attack as those who said they took no aspirin.

In the second part of the study, involving 10,542 patients, closer questioning may have increased reports of aspirin-taking among heart-attack victims. Still, those admitted for heart attacks were one-half as likely to be regular aspirin-takers as those who had not suffered heart attacks.

The extra information gathered in the special survey was then used to divide the patients into five groups with varying risk of heart attack. Such factors as smoking, coffee drinking, other drug use, and season of the year are known to increase or decrease heart-attack risk. Within each group, heart attacks were still roughly half as common among aspirin-takers as among persons who seldom took aspirin.

The BCDSP concluded that both first and recurrent non-fatal

heart attacks were less likely among persons who took aspirin regularly. But, the study warned, the evidence "fell far short of establishing that aspirin prevents" heart attacks. Still, the findings were termed "provocative," and controlled prospective studies were suggested.

In 1974, when the BCDSP retrospective aspirin-heart attack study was published, a prospective study was also published. Dr. Peter C. Elwood and fellow researchers in Cardiff, South Wales, compared the effect of aspirin to that of a placebo in reducing heart-attack risk. The group divided 1,126 men into a treated group, receiving one aspirin per day, and a control group, which got one placebo daily. Neither doctors nor patients knew who was in which group.

Elwood reported that he could not be certain his results were not by chance: either aspirin had an insignificant effect, or there were too few persons, studied for too short a time period. The inconclusive results: 8.3 percent of the aspirin group died, compared to 10.9 percent of the non-aspirin group.

One subsection of the study was statistically significant; among those whose treatment began within six weeks of their attack, only 7.8 percent of the aspirin group died, compared to 13.2 percent of the non-aspirin group.

The most recent completed prospective study of aspirin and heart-attack risk, published in 1976, was also inconclusive. The Coronary Drug Project Aspirin Study (CDPA), headquartered in Baltimore, found either the difference between aspirin and placebo was too small to detect, or else it had studied a small group too briefly. The National Heart Lung and Blood Institute supported the CDPA study.

Nevertheless, only 5.8 percent of the CDPA aspirin group died, compared to 8.3 percent of the placebo group. The researchers concluded their results were "suggestive of a therapeutic benefit" from taking aspirin. CDPA studied 1,529 men, most over fifty-five, receiving either three aspirin daily or a placebo, for up to twenty-eight months.

Ongoing Heart Studies

There are several major studies now underway in the United States to determine the relationship between aspirin use and heart-attack risk. The privately sponsored, nationwide, Baltimore-based Persantin-Aspirin Re-Infarction Study (PARIS) will follow 2,000 men and women for two years after the last one is registered. They will enter the program between two months and three years after their first attack. Incidence of death and heart attack will be noted in matched groups receiving aspirin, persantin, and a placebo.

In this and the other ongoing studies, strokes will be observed, but are not central to the study. Since stroke likelihood is lower than heart-attack likelihood, more persons would have to be studied for a longer period of time in order to obtain valid stroke prevention results.

Persons who have already had one heart attack were chosen for PARIS because their risk of a second attack is five times greater than the heart-attack risk of a person who has never had one. This reduces the number of persons and length of time needed for a study to produce statistically significant results.

The most ambitious ongoing study is the $17 million Aspirin Myocardial Infarction Study (AMIS), backed by the same federal agency, NHLBI, which supported the CDPA and Texas stroke studies. Actually, $17 million is only an estimate of the cost of observing 4,500 men and women across the country who have already had one attack. The selection of patients was completed in August, 1976; the study, based in Washington, D.C. will run until 1979, with results expected in 1980.

The study is randomized and double-blind; the treated group will get the equivalent of 1.5 aspirin tablets twice a day, while the control group will receive placebos of the same appearance. Men and women between the ages of thirty and seventy whose attacks occured between eight weeks and five years prior to the study were admitted.

AMIS will look for the two groups' relative death rate within three years of the attack, to see if aspirin has an effect. Results watched for will include death, death from heart attack, heart-at-tack rates in the control group, and stroke incidence in both groups. Side effects of long-term, low-dose aspirin use will also be recorded.

The co-ordinator of the study, Dr. William Friedewald, said the BCDSP, Elwood, and CDPA studies led to the decision to fund the AMIS study, as did the recent theoretical understanding of how aspirin might reduce the incidence of platelet plugs.

Dr. James Schoenberger, director of AMIS, talked to the author about the questions the study may answer and the ways in which its results will be examined:

> First, one has to ask the question, will you prevent someone who has already had a heart attack from having another one? Secondly, can you give this to individuals who have not had a heart attack? I don't think we'll have an answer to the second question. [The first] is all we are really trying to settle with this study.
>
> If the risks are not too high, and the benefits are good enough, then aspirin may have a very important role to play in intravascular clotting. But it is absolutely premature to discuss what I think are going to be the findings.
>
> Even if one percent who take it have a serious bleeding problem, and you only cut down the risk of heart attack by two percent, it is hardly worth it. These figures are only an example of what I mean by the cost-benefit ratio.

Take Aspirin for Prevention?

What can be done with the results of AMIS? Dr. Schoenberger speculated:

> I can't envision, even if aspirin proves to be success-ful in preventing recurring heart attacks, that we are go-

ing to go out and tell 100 million adults in the United States to take two aspirin a day. I just don't believe that is the way it is going to go.

If we prove it to be successful, we might tell people who have had heart attacks to take it, but I can't say we will do that until we know the answer. We might conceivably tell people who are at high risk of having a coronary, and these people can be identified, that they ought to take it.

I think a special study would have to be done to evaluate this. It would be more difficult than the previous one [AMIS] because it would take longer to get the answers, or it would take 4 to 5 times as many people.

The question of taking aspirin to prevent heart attacks was also posed to AMIS Co-ordinator, Dr. William Friedewald:

Why not give aspirin to everyone who has had a heart attack? When they have a serious problem, here's a drug with "no" side effects and no serious problems, if you rule out a few, why not give it to them?

No one has, routinely, over the long haul, studied people on low doses of aspirin. Unless we follow a large group of people for a reasonably long period of time, I don't think we know the toxicity. I think there are serious implications to telling someone they should take aspirin for the rest of their life to prevent a heart attack.

In an editorial in the *Journal of the American Medical Association*, the AMIS organizers suggested their study was "essential before a universal prescription for aspirin is inflicted on the public, who all to willingly seek easy answers to difficult problems."

The CDPA report also concluded there might be an increase in the "already massive use of aspirin, both via physician prescription and self-medication" because of its findings. The CDPA advised against aspirin-taking to prevent heart attacks because

109

"long-term use of any medication—including aspirin—should be undertaken only with provision for monitoring for long-term ill-effects."

There are physicians who disagree with the warnings of the medical estiablishment. Foremost among them is Dr. Lee Wood, a blood specialist in private practice in Covina, California, near Los Angeles. He is the most vocal of the medical critics of the go-slow approach to prescription of aspirin to prevent heart attacks.

Wood did not take his case to the public; instead he wrote for the doctors who read the prestigious British medical journal *Lancet*, in September, 1972. Prior to publication of any of the recent studies, he boldly proposed men over twenty and women over forty could take one aspirin tablet per day to reduce their chances of suffering from heart attack and stroke.

Research since then has done nothing to dissuade him, Wood said recently. He takes an aspirin tablet most days himself, while noting "it is hard to take medicine when you are feeling good."

In the *Lancet* article, he stated that, regardless of its effectiveness, aspirin treatment would be low-cost, the risks small at such doses, the theoretical basis sound, and the "possible benefits enormous."

Recently, Wood told the author that the new research findings indicate to him that as little as one aspirin tablet, twice a week, would affect about 50 percent of the platelets, on the average. This would cut even further aspirin's already low probability of side effects, he said.

Wood told us he was concerned about the results that will be reported from large-scale studies such as AMIS. "Their answer is going to be that aspirin doesn't do anything," he predicted. "The participants are going to read that aspirin may prevent a second heart attack, and the controls (those who are not being treated with aspirin) are going to go out and take it anyway."

The CDPA found, however, that only 6 percent of its participants admitted taking aspirin outside the program. It concluded a controlled study of aspirin could be performed among persons living normally.

Late in 1976, blood specialist Dr. Phillip Majerus, Washington University at St. Louis, wrote an editorial about aspirin as a heart-attack preventative for *Circulation*, an official journal of the American Heart Association. In it, he said aspirin's low rate of side effects made it an attractive anti-platelet drug.

"Even if the incidence of [heart attacks] is reduced only 10-20 percent," he wrote, "the [preventative] therapy of many 'normal' individuals could be justified."

Presently, it cannot be said with certainty whether regular aspirin-taking reduces a person's risk of heart attack and stroke. Even if the ongoing studies prove such a reduction, the determination of aspirin's effectiveness must be made on an individual basis. The physician and the patient must weigh the degree of risk and the level of adverse reaction to aspirin. No program of drug usage on a long-term basis should be entered into without the advice of a physician.

The author has discussed aspirin therapy with his own physician. His risk of heart attack is moderate; he is more than 10 percent over his ideal body weight, and one of his grandfathers died of a heart attack at age fifty-two, while one grandmother has severe high blood pressure. He suffers no discernible side effects from one aspirin tablet taken twice a week during the last year.

8

Aspirin's Future

The National Institute of Arthritis and Metabolic Diseases called aspirin "by far the most widely used and cheapest drug on earth, and one of the safest." That refers only to its present uses; aspirin may soon widen the already large gap between it and whatever medicine is second best, second less expensive, and second most widely available.

It has been more than 140 years since the first completely man-made medicine was introduced, 2,000 years since the first aspirin-like substance was used, and 78 years since aspirin itself became widely available. In all that time, no better drug than aspirin has been found for relief of pain without addiction, reduction of fever without side effects, and reduction of inflammation without serious disruption of bodily systems.

Individually and jointly, these three effects account for the vast majority of aspirin's present popularity. In any disease where these symptoms predominate, especially arthritis, aspirin is the drug physicians use first, to reduce symptoms while searching for causes. In the case of arthritis itself, aspirin halts the progress of the disease.

Aspirin is also popular because of its overall lack of serious side

113

effects. Drugs, as a rule, are either strong and specific in their effect, altering one system or affecting one organ; or they are general and weak, affecting several organs and systems. Specific drugs tend to produce more side effects, while general drugs tend be less effective. Aspirin is an exception to this rule: it has a strong effect on several systems, without producing significant side effects in most people at normal doses.

The present popularity of aspirin may just be the beginning. Studies now underway will check the preliminary finding that persons who take aspirin regularly are less likely to suffer from cardiovascular disease, blood clots after surgery, strokes or heart attacks. It has already been noted that persons who have heart attacks are less likely to have been regular aspirin users than those who have not had heart attacks. It remains to be proven that aspirin-takers are less likely to have heart attacks. If the latter proves true, treatment of heart-attack victims could be revolutionized, with as little as one or two aspirin tablets a day. Proof of this proposition is at least three years in the future.

Aspirin use may also skyrocket because of its effect on prostaglandins. The Upjohn Co., a major sponsor of PG research, has suggested the twenties were the decade of sex hormones, the thirties the decade of sulfa drugs, the forties antibiotics, the fifties polio vaccine and the sixties oral contraception. A company pamphlet contains the speculation that it takes "no crystal ball to foresee that the 1970s may well become the decade of the prostaglandins." PGs were not even in medical dictionaries as late as 1966; now three papers about them appear in medical journals every day. Aspirin is the safest drug that supresses prostaglandin production in humans. If the 1970s are the decade of prostaglandins, the 1980s may be the decade of aspirin's great leap forward.

There is gloom amid the joy, however, as concern grows amid doctors and the Food and Drug Administration about indiscriminate aspirin-taking. The *Journal of the American Medical Association* warned in a 1974 editorial of a growing number of products that contain aspirin without clearly implying the fact in their name.

The editorial said aspirin poses a risk for some, including those with ulcers, hemophelia, gout, or anti-coagulant therapy. "As the list [of aspirin-containing products] grows, the danger grows," the editorial stated.

The FDA, as part of its study of all over-the-counter drugs, has issued preliminary suggestions concerning aspirin, drafted by an advisory panel. Set to be finalized within the next two years, they include new warning labels about the dangers of overdose, and advise women in the last three months of pregnancy and persons with ulcers to avoid aspirin. The FDA advisory panel also tackled the thorny issue of multi-ingredient products—suggesting no OTC drug should have more than two active ingredients serving the same purpose. Use of the word "arthritis" in a product name may be banned.

The FDA rules are likely to result in some changes in the uses for which aspirin is advertised and the formulas in which it is available. They are not likely to result in any significant changes in public attitude toward the basic product, acetylsalicylic acid, or any major drop in daily usage.

Medical scientists will continue to search for more specific drugs that do aspirin's jobs better, with even fewer side effects. Now that they understand how aspirin works, the task has been made easier. It is not known at this time, however, if such drugs exist or can be economically produced. Possibly, drugs that do not work as well but have fewer side effects will take their place alongside already existing drugs that work better than aspirin in specific treatments, but which have more side effects.

Most promising of all is the possibility that, someday, "take two aspirins" may be a widespread prescription for reduction of the risk of heart attack.

Aspirin, the world's most widely used medical substance, is already best at what it does; soon, it may do more, winning an even broader role in medicine's chemical arsenal.

Appendix

A Partial Listing of Aspirin-containing Compounds Sold in the United States

Aidant
Alka Seltzer
Alprine
Amytal with Acetylsalic Acid
Anacin
Analgestine Forte
Anaphen
Anexsia D
Ansemco
Arthritis Strength Bufferin
Arthritis Pain Formula
As-Ca-Phen
Asalco No. 1
Asalco No. 2
Asco Solu-Caps

Asco Tablets
Ascodeen
Ascriptin
Aspergum
Asphac-G
Aspir-Code
Aspir-D Compound Capsules
Aspir-Phen
Aspirbar
Aspirin Aluminum
Aspirjen Jr. Tablets
Aspodyne
Axotal
ACA Capsules
APC

· ASPIRIN THERAPY ·

ASA Compound
ASA Enseals
ASA Preparation
B-A
Bayer Aspirin
Bexophene
Brogesic
Bufabar
Buff-a-Comp
Buffadyne
Bufferin
Buffinol
BC Tablets
Cama
Cap Capsules
Capathyn
Capron Capsules
Cefinal
Co-Ryd
Congespirin
Cope
Coralsone
Coricidin
Counterpain
Damason
Derfort
Derfule
Dolcin
Dolor
Doloral
Duradyne
Duragesic
Dynosal
Ecotrin
Empirin
Emprazil

Excedrin
Excedrin PM
Fiornal
Fizrin Powder
Gelsodyne
Goody's Headache Powder
Liquiprin
Marnal
Measurin
Midol
Milain
Niprin
Norgesic
Norwich Aspirin
Pabrin
PAC Capsules
Palgesic
Panodynes Analgesic
Percobarb
Percodan
Persistin
Phenacaps
Phenaphen
Phenodyne
Phensal
Presalin
Propoxyphene
Pyrihist Cold Capsules
Rhinex
Robaxisal
Rotense
Ryd Tablets
Sal-Fyne Capsules
Saleto
Salibar, Jr.
Salocol

Scrip-Dyne Compound
Sedagesic
Sine Aid
St. Joseph Aspirin
Stanback Powder
Stanback Tablets
Stanco
Stero–Darvon w/A.S.A.

Supac
Synalgos
Triaminicin
Trigesic
Valacet
Vanquish
4-Way

References

Ackerknecht, Erwin H. *Therapeutics*, New York: Hafner Press, 1973.

Altman, Raul, et. al. "Aspirin and prophylaxis of Thromboembolic complications," *J. Thor. and Card. Surg.*, July 1976.

American Medical Association. *AMA Drug Evaluations*, Acton, Ma.: Publishing Sciences Corp., 1973.

————. *Today's Health Guide*, Acton, Ma.: Publishing Sciences Corp., 1965.

American Pharmaceutical Association. *Brands, Generics, Prices and Quality*, Washington, D.C.: APA, 1971.

Anonymous, H.C. Wainwright & Co. Personal Interview, October 1976.

Anonymous (Manufacturing), Sterling Drug Inc.. Personal Interview, December 1976.

Anonymous (Press Relations), FDA Washington. Personal Interview, November 1976.

Arthritis Foundation. *About Gout*, New York.

————. *Arthritis: The Basic Facts*, New York. 1976.

————. *Arthritis Quackery*, New York.

————. *News Release*, June 9, 1976.

————. *Osteoarthritis*, New York.

————. *Rheumatoid Arthritis, A Handbook For Patients*, New York.

————. *The Truth about Aspirin for Arthritis*, New York.

————. *1975 Annual Report*, New York: 1975.

Aspirin Myocardial Infarction Study. "AMIS Protocol," Washington: October, 1975. Unpublished multilith or mimeograph.

Batterman, Robert C. "Comparison of Buffered and Unbuffered Acetylsalicylic Acid," *NEJM*, January 30, 1958.

Beaver, William T. "Mild Analgesics, A Review of their Clinical Pharmacology," *Am. J. Med. Sci.*, November 1965.

Black, William George. *Folk Medicine*, Glasgow: 1883.

Brendle, Thomas, and Unger, Claude. *Folk Medicine of the Pennsylvania Germans*, New York: Augustus M. Kelley, 1970.

Brooks, William J. *Facts About Aspirin*, New York: Sterling Drug, 1976.

Boston Collaborative Drug Surveillance Program. "Analgesic Consumption and Impaired Renal Function," *J. Chron. Dis.*, 1971.

————. "Drug Induced Deafness," *J. Am. Med. Assoc.*, April 23, 1973.

————. "Regular Aspirin Intake and Acute Myocaridal Infarction," *British Medical Journal*, March 9, 1974.

Capra, J. Donald, and Edmundson, Allen B. "The Antibody Combining Site," *Scientific American*, January 1977.

Chrisman, O. D. "Biochemical Aspects of Degenerative Joint Disease," *Clin. Ortho.*, May-June 1969.

————, et. al. "The Protective Effect of Aspirin against Degeneration of Human Articular Cartilage," *Clin. Ortho.*, May 1972.

————, and Snook, G.A. "Studies on the Protective Effect of Aspirin Against Degeneration of Cartilage," *Clin. Ortho.*, January 1968.

Coca-Cola Co. "The Chronicle of Coca-Cola since 1886," Atlanta: 1974. Privately published pamphlet.

Collier, H. O. J. "Aspirin," *Scientific American*, November 1963.

· REFERENCES ·

Coronary Drug Project Research Group. "Aspirin in Coronary Heart Disease," *J. Chron. Dis.*, February 8, 1976.

Craven, Lawrence L. "Prevention of Coronary and Cerebral Thrombosis," *Miss. Valley Medical J.*, September 1956.

Danhof, Ivan E. "Salicylate Analgesics and Fecal Blood Losses," Speech, April 26, 1972.

———, University of Texas. Personal Interview, January 1977.

Day, Arthur, UCSF Medical School. Personal Interview, December 1976.

DeKornfeld, Thomas, et. al. "A Comparative Study of Five Proprietary Analgesic Compounds," *J. Am. Med. Assoc.*, December 29, 1962.

Dixon, A. S., et. al., eds. *Salicylates*, London: J. & A. Churchill Ltd., 1963.

Done, Alan. "The Toxic Emergency: Acetaminophen," *Emergency Med.*, June 1975.

Donoso, E., and Haft, J.I., eds. *Thrombosis, Platelets, Anticoagulation*, New York: Stratton Intercontinental Book Corp., 1976.

Dreser, H. "The Pharmacology of Aspirin" (in German), *Pflugers Arch. Ges. Physiol.*, 1899.

Drug Therapy, "Aspirin: All the News Is Good," August 1974.

Duran-Reynals, M. L. *The Fever Bark Tree*, New York: Doubleday, 1946.

Dyken, Mark L., et. al. "Difference in the Occurrence of Carotid Transient Ischemic Attacks," *Stroke*, September-October 1973.

Earley, Kathleen. "The Truth about Aspirin," *Town and Country*, May 1977.

Ehrlich, George E. "Those Newer Antiarthritic Drugs—How They Work; How Well They Work," *Infectious Diseases*, November 1976.

Eichengrun, Arthur. Memoirs.

Evans, Geoffrey, McMaster University. Personal Interview, November 1976.

Falliers, Constantin J. "Familial Coincidence of Asthma, Aspirin Intolerance and Nasal Polyposis," *Ann. Allergy*, February 1974.

Farr, Richard S., National Jewish Hospital and Research Center. Personal Interview, November 1976.

Ferreira, S. H., and Vane, J. R. "Aspirin and Prostaglandins," *The Prostaglandins*, London: Plenum Press, 1974.

Fields, William S., "Controlled Trial of Aspirin in Cerebral Ischemia," January 1976. Manuscript.

————, and Hass, William K. *Aspirin, Platelets and Stroke*, St. Louis: Green, 1971.

————, University of Texas at Houston. Personal Interview, December 1976.

Freese, Arthur S. *Aspirin and your Health*, New York: Pyramid Books, 1974.

Friedewald, William, NHLBI AMIS Project Officer. Personal Interview, November 1976.

Friedman, Lawrence, NHLBI Medical Officer. Personal Interview, November 1976.

Friend, Dale G. "Aspirin: The Unique Drug," *Arch. Surg.*, June 1974.

FDA OTC Analgesic Panel. *Report*, Washington, D.C.: FDA, 1977.

————. *News Release*, July 7, 1977.

————. *Talk Paper*, October 26, 1977.

————. "Non-Prescription Medicines," Washington, D.C..

————. "Selecting your own Medicines," Washington, D.C.

————. "We Want You to Know about Prescription Drugs," Washington D.C.

————. "We Want You to Know about Labels on Medicines," Washington D.C.

FTC. (Press Relations), Washington, D.C. Personal Interview, November 1976.

Genton, Edward, et. al. "Platelet-inhibiting Drugs in the Prevention of Clinical Thrombotic Disease," *NEJM*, December 4, 1975.

————, et. al. "Platelet-inhibiting Drugs in the Prevention of Clinical Thrombotic Disease," *NEJM*, December 11, 1975.

————, et. al. "Platelet-inhibiting Drugs in the Prevention of Clinical Thrombotic Disease," *NEJM*, December 18, 1975.

Graedon, Joseph. *The People's Pharmacy*, New York: St. Martin's Press, 1976.

Griffenhagen, G., Hawkins, L. *Handbook of Non-Prescription Drugs*, American Pharmaceutical Association, Washington, D.C.: 1973.

Griffith, Valerie, *A Stroke in the Family*, New York: Delacorte Press, 1970.

Gross M., and Greenberg, L. *The Salicylates*, New Haven: Hillhouse Press, 1948.

Halpern, Lawrence M. "Treating Pain with Drugs," *Minnesota Medicine*, March 1974.

Harris, William, Harvard Medical School. Personal Interview, December 1976.

Hirsh, J., et. al., eds. *Platelets, Drugs and Thrombosis*, New York: S. Karger, 1975.

Hume, Michael, et. al. *Venous Thrombosis and Pulmonary Embolism*, Cambridge, Ma.: Harvard Press, 1970.

HEW. *News Release*, July 7, 1977.

Inglefinger, F. J. "The Side Effects of Aspirin," *NEJM*, May 23, 1974.

Internal Medicine News, "Routine Aspirin Use May Lower Rate of Myocardial Infarction," November 1, 1974.

Irwin, Susan, Dancer Fitzgerald Advertising. Personal Interview, November 1976.

Isomaki, H. A. "Aspirin and Myocardial Infarction in Patients with Rheumatoid Arthritis," *The Lancet*, October 14, 1972.

Jennings, J. J., et. al. "A Clinical Evaluation of Aspirin Prophylaxis of Thromboembolic Disease," *J. Bone and Joint Surg.*, October 1976.

Jick, Hershel, et. al. "A New Method for Assessing the Clinical Effects of Oral Analgesic Drugs," *Clin. Pharmacol. Ther.*, 1971.

J. Am. Med. Assoc. "Adverse Drug Interactions," 1972 Editorial.

———. "Aspirin and Myocardial Infarction: A New National Cooperative Trial," June 30, 1975.

———. "Aspirin by Prescription?," 1970.

Kakkar, V. V., and Jouhar, A. J. *Thromboembolism, Diagnosis, and Treatment*, London: Churchill Livingstone, 1972.

Kantor, Thomas. *Aspirin Revisted*, Chicago: American Rheumatism Association section of the Arthritis Foundation, June 9, 1976.

Kelley, Terry, Upjohn. Personal Interview, November 1976.

Kilbane, Paul, Murray Advertising. Personal Interview, November 1976.

Kolata, G. B. "Thromboxanes: The Power behind the Prostaglandins?," *Science*, November 21, 1975.

Lasagna, Louis. "Analgesic Drugs," *Am. J. Med. Sci.*, November 1961.

Lawson, David H. "Analgesic Consumption and Impaired Renal Function," *J. Chron. Dis.*, 1973.

Lee, Kwan-Hua, UCSF Medical School. Personal Interview, January 1977.

Levy, Gearhardt, SUNY Buffalo. Personal Interview, December 1976.

Levy, Joseph. Pacific Medical Center. Personal Interview, November 1976.

Levy, Micha. "Aspirin Use in Patients with Major Gastrointestinal Bleeding and Peptic Ulcer Disease," *NEJM*, May 23, 1974.

Majerus, Philip W. "Why Aspirin," *Circulation*, September 1976.

Meyer, J. S., et. al., eds. *Cerebral Vascular Disease, 6th International Conference, Salzburg*, St. Louis: C. V. Mosby Co., 1974.

————, ed. *Modern Concepts of Cardiovascular Disease*, New York: Spectrum Publications, 1975.

Miller, Russell R., and Jick, Hershel. "Acute Toxicity of Aspirin in Hospitalized Medical Patients." 1977. Manuscript.

Moertel, C. G., et. al. "A Comparative Evaluation of Marketed Analgesic Drugs," *NEJM*, April 13, 1972.

Moncada, S., et. al. "Prostaglandin Endoperoxides . . . inhibit(s) Platelet Aggregation," *Nature*, October 21, 1976.

Morrison, Margaret. "Medicine: Handle with Care," *FDA Consumer*, July-August 1976.

Mullen, W. R., Bates Advertising. Personal Interview, November 1976.

National Health Education Committee Inc. *Facts on the Major Killing and Crippling Diseases in the U.S.*, New York: 1971.

Nicolaides, A. N., ed. *Thromboembolism Etiology, Advances in Prevention and Management*, Baltimore: University Park Press, 1975.

Nies, Alan, Vanderbilt University. Personal Interview, November 1976.

NASA. *News Release*, July 16, 1968.

Plough, Inc. Various Pamphlets and News Releases.

Porter, Richard W. "A Modern Aspirin Plant," *Chemical Engineering*, March 1948.

Prescott, Frederick. *The Control of Pain*, New York: Thomas Y. Cromwell Co., 1964.

Product Management, "Breakdown of drug, cosmetic and toiletry sales," August 1976.

————, "1975 ad expenditures for health and beauty aids," July 1976.

Prostaglandins and Therapeutics, all issues, Upjohn Co., 1975-1977.

Rempen, F., Foltin, I. A., Bayer AG Leverkusen, Germany. Correspondence, December 1976.

Renney, J. T. G., et. al. "Prevention of Postoperative deep vein thrombosis," *British Medical Journal*, April 24, 1976.

Riegelman, Sidney, UCSF Medical School. Personal Interview, December 1976.

Rodman, Gerald P., ed. "Primer on the Rheumatic Diseases," J. of Am. Med. Assoc., April 30, 1973.

———, and Benedek, Thomas G. "The Early History of Antirheumatic Drugs," *Arthritis and Rheumatism*, March-April 1970.

Rouche, B. "Annals of Medicine, $CH_3CO_2C_6H_4CO_2H$," *New Yorker*, May 31, 1956.

Rumack, Barry, and Matthew, Henry. "Acetaminophen Poisoning and Toxicity," *Pediatrics*, June, 1975.

Russek, Henry I., and Zohman, Burton L. *Cardiovascular Therapy*, Baltimore: Williams & Wilkins Co., 1971.

Sadove, Max S., and Schwartz, Lester. "An Evaluation of Buffered Versus Nonbuffered Acetylsalicylic Acid," *Postgrad Med*, 1958.

Sahud, Mervyn. Testimony before the FDA, November, 1974.

Salzman, E. W., and Harris, W. H. "Prevention of Venous Thrombosis in Orthopaedic Patients," *J. Bone and Joint Surg.*, October 1976.

———, Harvard Medical School. Personal Interview, January 1977.

Scheinkey, P. "Cerebrovascular Diseases," *Stroke*, May-June 1977.

Schoenberger, James S., Aspirin Myocardial Infarction Study. Personal Interview, November 1976.

Science News, "How Aspirin Works," July 17, 1971.

Shuman, Mark, UCSF Medical School. Personal Interview, January 1977.

Silverman, Milton. *Magic In a Bottle*, New York: The MacMillan Co., 1948.

Slone, Dennis, et. al. "Aspirin and Congenital Malformations," *Lancet*, June 26, 1976.

Sterling Drug Inc. *Non-Prescription Pain Relievers: A Guide for Consumers*, New York: 1971.

————, *What Your Doctor Wants you to know about Aspirin*, New York: 1973.

Stone, Edmund. "On the Success of the Bark of the Willow in the Cure of Agues," *Philosophical Transactions*, April 25, 1763.

Strauss, Maurice B., and Welt, Louis G., *Diseases of the Kidney*, Boston: Little, Brown & Co., 1976.

Sutton, Ernest, and Soyka, Lester. "How Safe is Acetaminophen," *Clin. Pediatrics*, December 1973.

Tainter, Maurice L., and Ferris, Alice J. *Aspirin in Modern Therapy*, New York: Sterling Drug Inc., 1976.

Toole, James, F., and Patel, Aneel N. *Cerebrovascular Disorders*, New York: McGraw Hill, 1967.

The Upjohn Co. *Background Information: Prostaglandins: The New Frontier of Medical Science*, Kalamazoo, Mich.: Upjohn, 1972.

————. *The Prostaglandins*, Kalamazoo, Mich.: Upjohn, 1974¡

Van Tyle, W. K., Internal Analgeics Products. Pre-Publication Copy, American Pharmaceutical Association, December 1976.

Vane, John, Burroughs-Wellcome, England. Personal Interview, December 1976.

————. "Inhibition of PG Synthesis as a Mechanism of Action for Aspirin-like Drugs," *Nature New Biology*, June 1971.

Weiss, H. J. "Aspirin—A Dangerous Drug?," *J. Am. Med. Assoc.*, August 26, 1974.

————. Testimony before the FDA, November 1974.

————, Roosevelt Hospital, New York. Personal Interview, January 1977.

Winsor, Travis, and Hyman, Chester. *A Primer of Peripheral Vascular Diseases*, Philadelphia: Lea & Febiger, 1965.

Wolff, H. G. *Headache and Other Pain*, New York: Oxford University Press, 1972.

Wood, Lee. "Aspirin and Myocardial Infarction," *The Lancet*, November 11, 1972.

————, "Controlled Trials with Aspirin: Blindman's Bluff," *Modern Medicine*, April 1, 1976.

————, "Treatment of Atherosclerosis and Thrombosis with Aspirin," *The Lancet*, September 9, 1972.

————, Hematologist, Covina, Ca., Personal Interview, January 1977.

Woodbury, Carol, Herbist, Woodbury, Ct. Personal Interview, January 1977.

Index